Additional Praise for *A Path to Manhood*

"Paul Cumbo doesn't buy the cultural narrative that men are simple—and in stating this up front, he frees boys and young men to embrace their complexity. In *A Path to Manhood*, Cumbo empowers boys to create lives of meaning. A great book for teen and young adult males!" —**Jennifer L. W. Fink**, cohost of the *ON BOYS Podcast* and author of *Building Boys*

"With clarity, candor, and gentleness, Cumbo offers wise and down-to-earth counsel to young men navigating the unpredictable, challenging, and joy-filled paths of adolescence and young adulthood. *A Path to Manhood* is also a must-read for any educator or parent entrusted with the care of young men." —**Fr. Kevin O'Brien**, SJ, author of *The Ignatian Adventure* and *Seeing with the Heart*

"Cumbo intertwines the wisdom gained through his own life's journey with research across an array of pertinent fields in this timely, well-informed exploration of positive masculinity." —**Ann Holmquist**, EdD, vice president for mission, Loyola High School of Los Angeles

"Paul Cumbo has offered a great service to anyone involved in the adventure of raising boys—as parents, grandparents, teachers, coaches, or mentors. *A Path to Manhood* will offer dozens of conversation starters, inviting young men to think about the building blocks of a good life!" —**Tim Muldoon**, professor at Boston College and author of *Living Against the Grain*

T0356857

"The boy who learns to kindle and tend the fire will become the man who keeps us all warm. In *A Path to Manhood*, Paul Cumbo takes us on the spiritual and life journey that burns in each young man's heart and soul—his desire to be loved and purposeful in his home, his community, and his devotion to faith." —**Sean Kullman**, president of the Global Initiative for Boys and Men and coauthor of *Boys, A Rescue Plan*

"I was lucky to have Paul as a mentor in high school and witness firsthand his dedication to shaping men of character, compassion, and competence. Years later, *A Path to Manhood* opened my eyes to how much more there is to discover in my own journey as a father, husband, and artist. I encourage other guys to read this inspiring book. Anyone with a son, husband, or brother will also gain an illuminating perspective." —**Ian Harding**, father, star of *Pretty Little Liars*, and author of *Odd Birds*

"A must-read for every guy on the path to Christian manhood." —**Mark E. Thibodeaux**, SJ, author of *God's Voice Within*

"*A Path to Manhood* shows young men that they are not alone. Connection—with others and themselves—is key, and reading this book will teach young men that it is a necessary part of their life path." —**Dr. Brigid Vilardo Lyons**, PhD, licensed psychologist

"Cumbo, matching challenge with encouragement, calls on today's guys to cultivate an authentic masculine spirit and to strengthen it by traveling a path of honor, love, service, gratitude, faith, and courage." —**Heidi M. Weiker**, MSSA, stress resilience specialist and co-owner of Spherica

A PATH TO MANHOOD
Encouragement and Advice for Young Men

PAUL CUMBO

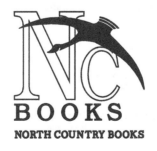

BOOKS
NORTH COUNTRY BOOKS

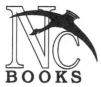

BOOKS
NORTH COUNTRY BOOKS

An imprint of The Globe Pequot Publishing Group, Inc.
64 South Main Street
Essex, CT 06426
www.globepequot.com

Distributed by NATIONAL BOOK NETWORK

British Library Cataloguing in Publication Information Available

Library of Congress Cataloging-in-Publication Data

Names: Cumbo, Paul, author.
Title: A path to manhood : encouragement and advice for young men / Paul Cumbo.
Description: Essex, CT : North Country, [2025]
Identifiers: LCCN 2024034691 (print) | LCCN 2024034692 (ebook) | ISBN 9781493089000 (paperback ; alk. paper) | ISBN 9781493089017 (ebook)
Subjects: LCSH: Young men—Conduct of life. | Men—Identity. | Adulthood.
Classification: LCC BJ1671 .C86 2025 (print) | LCC BJ1671 (ebook) | DDC 158.1084/21—dc23/eng/20241025
LC record available at https://lccn.loc.gov/2024034691
LC ebook record available at https://lccn.loc.gov/2024034692

♾️™ The paper used in this publication meets the minimum requirements of American National Standard for Information Sciences—Permanence of Paper for Printed Library Materials, ANSI/NISO Z39.48-1992.

Contents

Caminante, no hay camino,
se hace camino al andar.

Walker, there is no road,
the road is made by walking.

—A<small>NTONIO</small> M<small>ACHADO</small>

"Proverbios y Cantares **XXIX**"
Campos de Castilla (1912)

Machado, A. *Border of a Dream.* Port Townsend, WA: Copper Canyon Press, 2004.

Foreword

Luke Russert

THE EVIDENCE IS OVERWHELMING, whether analytical, empirical, scientific, or anecdotal. Young men are at a crisis point. They have dropped out of the labor market and fallen behind on their education. Addiction is rampant, and suicide rates are on the rise. Why is this?

There are a multitude of reasons. Some will say young men have fallen victim to our digital times: they're caught in an endless wave of social media, video games, and pornography, manipulated by disingenuous actors profiteering off their impressionable anxiety. They are being taught to be angry and exhibit false bravado for political purposes. Others will say a lack of fathers in the home has contributed and the common cliché "men no longer know how to be men" holds true—in essence, a new modern society is forcing them to abandon their masculinity. I do not subscribe fully to either theory, but I do feel there's a sad reality that has set in—not enough people care about our young men in America.

Too many say that men have been so privileged for so many generations that their plight is simply a correction that was set to happen once society evolved. Another subset wants men to revert back to a time when women were considered subservient and minority rights were few.

Where are young men to turn when, upon reflection, they're being told that everything is all their fault or that being hyperaggressive and invulnerable is their duty as a man?

I hope they turn to this book.

Paul Cumbo admits he does not have all the answers. Young men are a diverse group, and some are further along in the maturation process than others. But what he does have is an optimistic and uplifting worldview, born out of years of helping to shape minds.

As Paul says, "I'm not a doctor, a priest, a psychologist, or a therapist. But here's who I am: I'm one of five brothers. I'm a husband, fifteen years into my marriage. I'm a father to two sons and a daughter. I'm a writer, coach, and mentor with a handful of letters after my name. I'm an entrepreneur and small business owner. Mostly, though, I'm a teacher."

This makes Paul relatable. He's brilliantly direct and understandable. In *A Path to Manhood*, he does what the most effective communicators and teachers do—meet young men on their level in language they can understand. Whether it's talking about the need for companionship, being open, establishing emotional connections, taking care of health—mental and physical—or just embracing vulnerability, Paul teaches truly valuable lessons of life.

I was fortunate to grow up with great parents and mentors, especially a father who taught me the intrinsic value of "You're always loved but you're never entitled." That has helped me a lot in life. So did the coaches who taught me to dig down, persevere, and give it my all, and the importance of showing up. But one thing was missing from my formation as a man—vulnerability. For many years, I did not know how to ask for help, especially after my father passed away. I did not want to be a burden, and I felt I could get by on my own. I was lost and adrift. I threw myself into hard work, spirited revelry, or long travel. Anything to mask the pain of grief or discouragement. Thankfully I realized that to move forward, I had to open myself up and grab hold of that helping hand.

This book is that hand. Its pages remind us it is okay to lean on others and learn from them. We should; we need to. It's a lesson for men, young or old. I thank Paul Cumbo for writing it and look forward to the day I can hopefully gift it to my son.

Luke Russert
Washington, DC, Summer 2024

CHAPTER ONE

Making Your Path

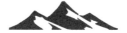

A LITTLE BOY LIVED BY A STREAM. He spent summer days exploring the woods, playing hide-and-seek with his friends and hunting for crawfish in the cool water under the rocks. One morning, as he sat on the bank of the creek waiting for his buddies, he began stacking stones. Soon he had a small tower, and he found that he was enjoying the building process. Sensing the need for more strength, he began mixing mud and gravel to make thick mortar, which he layered carefully among the stones. Now his tower took on a pleasing symmetry. His friends had not shown up at the usual time to play, but he hardly noticed.

The boy was focused on his tower.

At lunchtime, as he devoured his peanut butter and jelly sandwich and chugged a cold glass of milk, he resolved to build the tallest tower *ever*. He spent the afternoon crafting his masterpiece. Sweat, mosquitoes, and chafed hands didn't slow him down. When the project grew taller than the boy, he built a scaffold out of rocks and logs. He kept at it until the tower was a thing of beauty nearly twice his height. He even found a sparkling piece of quartz in the dirt around the stream, which he decided to use as the capstone. Carefully, he climbed, balancing and stretching, to place the quartz on top.

That's when the scaffolding shifted—just a bit, but just enough.

Losing his balance, he fell straight into the tower. It toppled into the creek with a thunderous splash. A seething frustration boiled up from within him, and before he knew it, he was crying the hot, bitter tears that boys his age cry. Then he heard someone approaching, a new neighbor boy he'd seen moving in but hadn't met yet. Quickly, he wiped his tears away. He was too old to be seen crying, of course.

"Hi," said the new kid, sitting down next to him. "Cool bridge! Mind if I help?"

The first boy looked at the line of stones spanning the stream, marveling now at the bridge-building possibilities that lay sprawled before him amid the ruins of his tower. "Yeah. Sure," he said. And with that, the two set themselves to work. Only after they began placing stones did they remember to tell each other their names.

Before long, the two boys had shored up the rocks to form a sturdy bridge across the stream. Stopping to rest in the shade for a while, they noticed that the bridge was also acting as a dam and that the deepening water behind it formed a pool. Hot and sweaty from their work, they peeled off their shirts and jumped in, splashing and laughing.

After their swim, they sat on the bridge, drying off in the hot sun. That's when they noticed the fish swimming around in the pool that had formed. The boys ran home, got their fishing poles, baited their hooks, and cast the lines into the pool. They didn't catch anything, but it hardly mattered. As evening set in and dinnertime approached, they traded high-fives and see-ya-laters.

That night, as the boy's mother tucked him into bed, she asked him what he'd been so busy doing all day.

"I built a bridge. And I made a new friend. And we went swimming. And we went fishing."

"Sounds like a good day," she said as she turned out the light.

"Yeah. Really good," he said, and went to sleep.

BE OPEN TO NEW POSSIBILITIES

Stories can be fictional, like that one, and still tell the truth.

That story is a reflection of a part of my life, and maybe yours, too. Because sometimes we learn that what we thought should be a tower—what we *willed* to be a tower—could just as well serve as a bridge. Maybe, in fact, we figure out that it would serve even better as a bridge instead, despite our . . . well, "towering" aspirations.

This book is going to ask you to be open to the idea that your building materials—the things that make you *you*—can be used for more than one thing, and that the events in your life might have more meaning, or different meanings, than you've initially understood.

That your life has purpose and is full of possibilities you may not yet have considered.

That you can be a man of virtue—the kind of man people genuinely respect—if you're willing to work at it.

If you're willing to make your own path as you go.

WALKER, THERE IS NO ROAD

Sometimes a single word can make a big difference. Look at the cover of this book for a second. I chose the title *A Path to Manhood*. It's not *The Path to Manhood*. That's only a one-word difference, but it's a big one: "a path" versus "the path." *The* path suggests there's only one prescribed road to growing up from boyhood to manhood. That's not the case. You've got to make your own path. That's what this book is about.

You might have noticed the excerpt from a poem by the Spanish writer Antonio Machado near the front of the book. Machado suggests that not only do we have to travel through life, but that we also must make our own path: "Walker, there is no road / the road is made by walking." It sounds even better in Spanish: "*Caminante, no hay camino / se hace camino al andar.*"[1] Making your path is a messy thing, but making a good path is a noble undertaking for any young guy.

I'm guessing you care about the direction of your path. Otherwise, why would you read this? We hear about how "life is a journey" all the time. It's a cliché. Know what, though? Often, clichés only get to be clichés because they're so damn true.

"Not All Those Who Wander Are Lost"

Throughout this book, I'm going to encourage you to make your own path. But that doesn't mean you have to create it from scratch, or that you can't ever travel established routes, or even follow the example of others. Making your path doesn't always mean creating new roads—it just means making your own decisions about where *you* will go.

Truth is, that's bound to involve some wandering. That isn't the same as wandering *aimlessly*. If we don't know what we're aiming for, it's difficult to pursue it. Dr. Jordan Peterson, a well-known psychologist and author, has written eloquently about aim. In his book, *12 Rules for Life: An Antidote to Chaos*, he suggests that "we cannot navigate, without something to aim at, and while we are in this world, we must always navigate."[2] It's tough to climb a mountain if we don't know where the top is. Even if we never end up reaching it, we still need to know the point we're aiming for if we're going to forge a path in the right direction. Consider a famous line from J. R. R. Tolkien's *The Fellowship of the Ring*, "Not all those who wander are lost," which we first encounter amid other verses in Gandalf's letter to Frodo. Later, we learn the poem was written by Bilbo about Aragorn, a man who did plenty of wandering—but certainly not aimlessly.[3]

So how do we wander with purpose? How do we allow ourselves the freedom to make our own paths—including some messy detours—without getting lost? I think we can look to the advice of Dr. Viktor Frankl. Frankl, a psychiatrist and Holocaust survivor, articulated an important idea in his seminal work

Man's Search for Meaning. In his preface to the 1992 edition, Frankl wrote:

> *Don't aim at success—the more you aim at it and make it a target, the more you are going to miss it. For success, like happiness, cannot be pursued; it must ensue, and it only does so as the unintended side-effect of one's dedication to a cause greater than oneself or as the by-product of one's surrender to a person other than oneself. Happiness must happen, and the same holds for success: you have to let it happen by not caring about it. I want you to listen to what your conscience commands you to do and go on to carry it out to the best of your knowledge. Then you will live to see that in the long run—in the long run, I say!—success will follow you precisely because you had* forgotten *to think of it.*[4]

Frankl's words here are very freeing. They allow us—in fact, they challenge us—to make our own path, but in the service of some meaningful, long-term aim. Frankl suggests we should let go of a focus on our own success, and even our own happiness, and that in doing so we will find both. In a sense, he calls us to wander on a path-making journey—but with purpose. Because, well, "not all those who wander are lost."

The Depth and Complexity of Masculinity

As the subtitle suggests, I wrote this book to offer encouragement and advice to young men. By that I mean teenagers and guys in their early to mid-twenties—a group that could fairly be described as "emerging men." When I do presentations at schools or for other groups of emerging men, I use the Grand Canyon as a metaphor for a guy's interior life. The Grand Canyon is deep. Its layered, striated rock faces reveal remarkable geologic complexity that undergoes constant change, compelled by powerful forces of nature. Currents in the river formed some of the striata over time—currents often invisible to most people and hidden deep below the surface of the surrounding landscape. For most boys and men, the complexity of our interior life is often hidden. Male waters run deep in the chasms of our hearts.

Masculinity is just as complex. I don't buy the cultural narrative that men are simple. Our understanding of masculinity shouldn't be limited to the narrow, reductive definition characterized by traditionally rugged masculine norms. At the same time, we should embrace traditional masculine norms like strength, resilience, self-sufficiency, courage, loyalty, and grit. They shouldn't be underestimated, frowned upon, or labeled as outdated. The world needs strong men just as much as it needs strong women. If strong people aren't around, weak people will take charge. That doesn't go well.

But strength comes in many forms, and masculinity is complex enough to include a range of temperaments, attitudes, and sexual orientations. One need only study history to come to this realization. Hopefully, this open-minded perspective will be apparent throughout the course of this book, and I would like to think what I've written here will be relevant to any young man who reads it. If you're drawn to fast cars, play baseball, and get turned on by pretty girls, this book is for you. Same if you're not into sports and would rather play Dungeons & Dragons on a Friday night than go to a party. If you find yourself more attracted to the other guys on your football team than you are to the girls in the cheerleading squad—or just as much, anyway—this book is for you, too. I'll stop there with the hypotheticals; they could go on forever. And that's because I haven't written this for a "certain kind of guy." I've written this for *all* guys, at an age when they're still figuring out who they are and what kind of men they want to be.

This is also a response to a cultural narrative that too often, and too simplistically, casts a negative light on teenage guys and young men. Just getting this book published is illustrative of that cultural narrative. Several industry experts told me there's no way guys in their late teens and early twenties would sit down and read a book like this. Beyond that, the story told by much of our media is an alarmist tale of boy crisis after boy crisis. At best, boys and young men are hapless, listless, or lazy; at worst, they are inherently malevolent, predatory, and violent.

I'd like to think my view—which has come about from experience and over time—is balanced. I have worked with thousands of teenage guys, and I've mentored a lot of them into their twenties—some even beyond that. On one hand, I have seen some young men do horrible things to themselves and to others. I've seen dishonesty, depravity, mendacity, cruelty, addiction, abuse, and even criminal behavior. It has occasionally left me feeling hopeless, angry, betrayed, and cynical. But anyone who's been alive for a while knows that's only part of the story. The truth is, everyday life tells us that kindness outweighs cruelty, decency is more common than indecency, and most people, most of the time, try to do the right thing. That applies to men and women alike, but when it comes to teenage boys and young men, our culture portrays an incomplete picture. I believe there's a particular need for more exploration of male complexity, emotional and intellectual depth, and potential. This book will pose tough questions and explore complex ideas.

There's also a need for a clear call to virtue. I've never met a guy who didn't want, deep down, to be the best version of himself. That takes work. We have to *strive* for it, always. That's what this book is calling you to do. Aim. Strive. Build your path in pursuit of it.

That's how you make a good path, even when you wander.

What This Book Is and Isn't

Who am I to call you to strive for virtue?

First, I'll tell you who I'm not: I'm not a doctor, a priest, a psychologist, or a therapist. But here's who I am: I'm one of five brothers. I'm a husband, fifteen years into my marriage. I'm a father to two sons and a daughter. I'm a writer, coach, and mentor with a handful of letters after my name. I'm an entrepreneur and small business owner.

Mostly, though, I'm a teacher. Teaching takes many forms. This book is being published during my twenty-third year in the high school classroom. But I also spent about half those years coaching crew, teaching teenage guys the rhythms and poetry of rowing—helping them craft the strength, endurance, agility, and mental precision that yields speed on the water. I have led many service learning trips with students to places near and far, immersive experiences that challenge us to step out of our comfort zone and wrestle with big questions about the world. I cofounded a company that leads multiple retreats each year at our campus in the Dominican Republic, mostly for young adults.

Mentoring former students as they've entered the often confusing and perilous years of their early to mid-twenties keeps me aware of how hard that stage of life can be. Through all of this I've found a genuine and near-constant joy in the work, which, of course, is really all about people. This brings me to my most important qualification for teaching and for writing this book: being a guy. Being human, just like you. Growing up is a struggle, and I've been there.

I want to be clear on something: This isn't a political book. I don't have a political agenda. I don't belong to a political party, and I don't vote on party lines. I think the recent rise of identity politics has been a damaging influence on the fabric of our society, and responsibility for that damage lies with those who embrace the kind of reductive, zero-sum ideologies we've seen spring like weeds from *both* ends of the political spectrum.

My political centrism, then, reflects my belief in balance, a motif you'll encounter often in these pages. I think most of the currents of what matters most in our lives run deeper than the often-shallow waters of politics. I also think most people are of a similar mind. The center is called the "silent majority" for a reason.

I'm a practicing Roman Catholic, and I'm the product of Jesuit education at the high school, college, and graduate school level. (The Jesuits are an order of Catholic priests and brothers founded about five hundred years ago, and they have a big focus on education. I've been working at Jesuit high schools for boys for my entire career.) My insights on marriage and relationships are grounded, primarily, in my experience as a husband and father in a traditional marriage. What's here represents my own opinions and beliefs about how guys can strive for virtue on the journey to manhood. You might disagree with some of what I say. That's okay. Intelligent men can respectfully disagree on things. People don't have to agree on everything to learn from each other. Just keep an open mind and think for yourself.

COURAGE FOR THE JOURNEY

I wrote this book to challenge and encourage you at the same time. In fact, much of my encouragement lies in the form of challenges—challenges to *stop* doing some things, *keep* doing others, and *start* doing others. Within the word "encourage" lies another: "courage." To encourage means to bolster someone's courage. To support what they are undertaking. To affirm the effort and the person making it. Tough undertakings involve discomfort, suffering, or even considerable danger. These are things that demand courage—so we need encouragement. You might have noticed that our culture is very vocal when it comes to encouraging girls and women. That's a good thing. But at the same time, I don't hear the same messages being passed down to boys and men. In fact, I think our culture has in many ways turned a blind eye to the struggles of boys and men. That's not a good thing.

Calling this out can get you in trouble, though.

Well, I'm willing to take that risk—because everyone needs encouragement. Yes, even boys and young men. Yes, even *difficult* boys and young men.

Years ago, I had this tenth-grade student that nobody liked—let's call him Joe. Joe was lazy, a little sneaky, and a little bit nasty, too. Something happened halfway through sophomore year, and he tried to turn things around. He stopped being a jerk, and his grades began to improve. They were Cs, not As, but that was a big climb from the Ds and Fs he'd been earning.

But instead of encouraging him, I confess I sometimes joined in the snarky faculty room chatter about Joe, joking about how long it would be before he slipped back into his old habits. I never made an effort to affirm the changes he was making.

I finally caught up with him the following year, and we had a good talk. I learned some stuff about his life that helped me understand him. The kid was fighting some battles I didn't know about. I realized I'd made too many assumptions.

I changed my tune. I encouraged him. Better late than never, right?

Look, we don't need to give out participation trophies for doing what's expected. That said, we all need encouragement, because confronting life takes . . . well, courage.

A CALL TO VIRTUE

What's virtue? Virtue means making a habit of doing the right thing. At its root is the Latin word *vir*, meaning "man." Taken a step further closer to the word we know, the Latin *virtus* means "masculine strength" or, more roughly translated, "manliness."

This doesn't refer only to physical strength. Nor is it exclusive to men—certainly, virtues are embodied by women! The connection here is to "mankind," as in "humankind." But for us as men, it suggests that deep within the core of our humanity—part of which is our masculinity—lies the potential to do the right thing. If you think about it, that's both challenging *and* encouraging.

I cling to that encouragement, because I know I'm a mess. I have all kinds of daily struggles. Moral struggles, ethical struggles. Struggles to be a better husband, father, son, brother, teacher, and friend.

You have some struggles, too.

I wrote this book because I believe you and I are capable of being better men today, tomorrow, and beyond. That we have the capacity, if we can match it with sufficient will, to make a good path. That we can make the climb. The Greek term *arete* refers, literally, to a sharp precipice of a mountain. It's the jagged peak piercing the clouds. But it also means excellence. If we aim for the knife-edge, the pinnacle, the *arete*, we can achieve virtue. I think our best chances lie with holding each other accountable, encouraging and learning from one another as we travel.

I agree with Machado. *No hay camino.* There is no universal road, and we each have to make our own path. But nobody said we have to do it alone.

So, let's walk together for a while.

CHAPTER TWO

Not a Straight Line

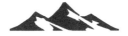

THE AMERICAN PHILOSOPHER AND WRITER Ralph Waldo Emerson, in his well-known 1841 essay "Self-Reliance," suggested that "the voyage of the best ship is a zigzag line of a hundred tacks. See the line from a sufficient distance, and it straightens itself to the average tendency." Emerson was referring to the fact that for a ship to sail into the wind, it has to tack—that is, switch back and forth on courses that catch the headwind at an angle. Close up, it hardly looks like efficient progress. Zoom out far enough, though, and those many detours blur themselves to "the average tendency."

Your path is going to zig and zag, but in the end, looking back, what will be its "average tendency"? Not perfect. But hopefully, one toward virtue. Hopefully, one marked by excellence. It's also worth considering this idea in terms of how we view the paths of people we admire. When we look at the trajectory of the paths traveled by people who impress us, we might not see the many zigs and zags. Unless we take the time to look very closely, we might be tempted to think those lines were pretty straight, without deviation. That's a mistake, because we tend to compare our own messy paths with ideals that just don't match reality. I think you'll see this as you get older—people you once put on a pedestal come into sharper focus, and you see that almost everyone's path is a little more complicated than it might have appeared from a distance. But here's the thing: that doesn't necessarily make them any less impressive. In fact, you might find that it makes them *more* admirable.

Perfection versus Excellence

At the close of the previous chapter, I explained the dual meanings of the Greek word *arete*. Consider the literal meaning for a moment: the precipice of a mountain. Getting there might involve a long, difficult, dangerous trek. You need know-how, strength, endurance, agility, and no small amount of perseverance. First and foremost, you need a *desire* to get there. A strong one. A *genuine* one. Because it isn't easy, so if the desire isn't really there, well, it probably isn't going to happen. You're apt to give up, go home, and have a sandwich instead.

But *arete* isn't only about mountaintops. It also means excellence. Not perfection, but excellence in the sense of trying to live up to one's *full* potential in any aspect of life. Specifically, it refers to excellence in the context of moral virtue—something we'll take a look at soon.

There's a big difference between perfection and excellence. I'm not going to achieve perfection, and you're not either, because we're human. Besides, why be perfect? Perfection would mean we couldn't improve. That's actually pretty discouraging. I don't want to think that, in this life, there's a place we can get to where nothing better lies beyond. No higher achievement possible? No improvement to be made? Who would want that? What the heck would we do? I am always inspired more by the quest for *arete*—for excellence.

Perfection is unattainable. But isn't excellence another prospect altogether? Isn't excellence what we achieve when we are really, truly engaging our best effort at something—even though we know we can't reach perfection? I think so. Why?

Maybe because it *isn't* driven by fear. See, I believe people obsessed with perfection are often driven too much by fear of failure. This fear is a powerful motivator, but it's not a good prospect for the long haul. It's too exhausting. When people come to understand that they aren't going to achieve perfection, they accept that failure is an essential part of the process.

Instead of fear, people aiming for excellence are driven by the motivation that comes from gradual improvement. They know that on the quest for excellence, minor improvements are major successes. This is different from the quest for perfection, on which minor improvements barely register (in fact, they might actually discourage us because they're so, well, minor). People aiming for excellence know the truth: life is a slow, steady climb, and each step matters. And the toughest part, sometimes, is simply to keep going.

Let me tell you a story about that.

On Being a Mess

I coached a kid I'll call Sam. (In some cases, I'll be using fictional names like this to refer to real people to help ensure their privacy.) After Sam got in big trouble midway through high school, he was depressed. He was seeing a counselor, but we'd connected as coach and athlete, so his parents asked if I'd come over to talk to him. As we walked around his neighborhood, hands buried in our pockets, he struggled to find the words to say what he was feeling. After several minutes of silence, he stopped and looked me in the eye and asked, "Why am I such a mess, Coach?"

Sam had known his share of trouble. I'd met him on the first day of our rowing team's preseason training camp his freshman year. He was rambunctious, rebellious, and angry, with hair as unruly as his personality. Sometimes his eyes would seethe with fiery anger; other times they seemed cold and distant. You didn't need a degree in psychology to sense this kid had been through some stuff.

I pushed him hard at practice, and I soon realized he craved the discipline and structure our team provided. He did well that year, making competitive boats. (Rowing teams are often large, with several dozen athletes, but a "crew" or "boat" refers to the lineup of athletes—rowers and coxswain, or pilot, placed in a particular racing shell to race in a specific event, typically designated by age and weight class. This placement is a competitive prospect, with the top performers grouped together in the most competitive boats.) The harder I pushed Sam, the more he responded. We bonded the way athletes and coaches often do. I came to know his complicated family story. I was sympathetic, but I tried hard not to let my sympathy show. He despised being babied, and he didn't want to be let off the hook. He wanted to be held accountable. He didn't want special treatment. I admired that.

When I'd see him in the hallways during the school day, I'd stay on him, nixing his shenanigans before they could get him off track. I learned a lot about Sam and the demons he wrestled with. We had honest talks, one on one and with various counselors. A couple years in, it seemed Sam had turned a corner. While he could still be trouble, he'd matured. But soon things fell apart, and a series of bad decisions exhausted his "second" chances at school. As I looked at Sam during our walk around his neighborhood, tears welling up in my own eyes, I felt the messiness of life for sure. "We're all a mess," I said. "But don't forget that you matter."

He nodded, and we walked back to his house. As he headed inside, I waved to his parents. Alone in the car, I cried on the drive home, because I wasn't sure he believed what I'd told him. And, of course, I could remember a time in my life when I might not have believed it myself.

We Matter

I have a fundamental belief that we matter; as such, the path that we make matters. There was a time in my life, around age nineteen, when my own life seemed so messy that I was pretty sure everything was arbitrary and meaningless. Looking back, I now understand that I was conflating messiness with meaning-lessness. I was under the mistaken impression that if something was messy and imperfect, it didn't have much value.

I couldn't have been more wrong.

As a result of this limited understanding, the path I walked between late adolescence and my early twenties was in many ways a dark, dangerous stretch. I'm lucky to have emerged from it intact, and that was thanks to the guidance and mentoring of some wise people who really looked out for me.

They helped me understand that I matter.

My work with boys and young men in the decades since then has shown me that many young guys—guys like Sam, for example—find themselves in a place where they don't believe their lives have genuine worth. Or, at best, they're unsure if they do. The reasons vary. Sometimes it comes from having failed at something like school, sports, a job, or a relationship. For me, it had to do with a specific failure after high school and the regrets that followed in its wake. I'll tell you more about that later.

But there are many different reasons why guys struggle to believe they matter. Sometimes, this lack of a sense of self-worth takes root in a difficult upbringing, perhaps with a troubled, neglectful, or even abusive relationship with a parent or other family member. Often, guys question their self-worth because they haven't reached personal, professional, or relational milestones they think they should have by a certain age—I see this more often with guys in their twenties.

For some teens and young men, coming to terms with their sexuality is a frightening struggle that causes them to question their fundamental goodness and worth. Our culture is more open-minded than it used to be—but that doesn't make things easy for anyone navigating the path of his emerging sexuality, especially a gay or bisexual teen who might be experiencing shifting feelings and attractions that leave him feeling confused, ashamed, or alone.

Many guys struggling with an addiction—whether to substances like drugs or behaviors like porn use or gambling—despise themselves for it. There are so many forces that can cause teen guys and young men to feel hopeless, and that hopelessness can sometimes lead to terrible outcomes. One need only look at the rising rates of suicide among guys to see that.

Maybe some of what I've described here relates to you. Maybe you've questioned your own self-worth for one reason or another. And even if you haven't had to wrestle with such heavy issues, you've at least had some tough days by the time you're old enough to be reading this book.

It's so important to know that you matter.

That your life, and the path you travel, has genuine worth.

To be encouraged.

We matter, in the big scheme of things. That's my attitude toward life, and it's fair to say it informs everything written in this book. My disposition is grounded in faith—and it's been a hard-earned faith, not a blind adherence to religious dogma. I believe our lives have genuine value because I believe we have the spark of the divine in us—that we were each made, intentionally and lovingly, by God. That's a foundational principle of my Catholic faith.

There's a story from the Christian Gospels that I really like because it shows this so well. You can find it in a couple places: Matthew 8 or Luke 7. A Roman centurion—a guy who would not exactly be considered an amigo of the early Christians—approaches Jesus and asks him to heal his servant. The first thing the centurion says to Jesus is, "I am not worthy to have you come under my roof, but just say the word and my servant shall be healed."

The soldier knows he's a mess, just like you and me, and he has the humility to acknowledge it. But he also has faith in the love Jesus has become known for, and he has the humility to ask for help. This story is the basis for an important prayer before Communion during the Catholic Mass: "Lord, I am not worthy that you should enter under my roof, but only say the word and my soul shall be healed." That's my favorite part of the Mass.

That's what Christianity tells us: we're each a mess, but God loves us anyway—and that makes sense, after all, since that's how we were made! But you don't have to believe in God, per se, to believe life has genuine value. Let's say you don't believe in God, or you aren't sure if you do. Okay. It's good enough that you believe in *something*—or at least, that you *want* to. I mean, if you didn't believe life mattered, you wouldn't bother reading a book like this, right? But here you are reading it.

Another way of thinking about it is in mathematical, economic terms. Given the sheer volume of space, the fact that you and I exist at all—moreover as sentient, sovereign, self-aware, intelligent beings capable of pondering our own existence—is a mathematical improbability of such proportions that it's downright miraculous. Using basic principles of economics (supply and demand, scarcity yielding value), we realize that we are in such short supply compared to the space we inhabit that our value is astronomical.

Pun intended, of course.

So if we matter so much, why do we suffer so much?

SUFFERING

Despite my firm belief in how valuable and significant each of us is, I know I'm a mess. I wonder if maybe you are, too. It's not hard to know we're messy. Because of the suffering, right?

Life is full of suffering. Pain is one of the first things we learn, and it's wired into our limbic system—one of the most primitive, ancient parts of our brain. Fight or flight—the two instinctive responses most deeply embedded in our neural networks—are based on the perception of, response to, and avoidance of pain, whether physical or emotional.

23

If you've been walking your path for a while, even if you're among the most fortunate guys on the planet, you've known your share of pain. It's one of the things we have in common with everyone else on the planet. We've all scraped our knees on the sharper parts of the earth. Some have experienced much worse than that.

The Greek word *pathos* is very interesting. It means "suffering." But it also means "experience." Kind of cool that the same word means both things, right? Then again, it makes perfect sense. We tend to accumulate the most valuable life experiences when we suffer, either a little or a lot. We *empathize* and *sympathize* with people because our experience of suffering allows us to relate to theirs. Sam's *pathos*—his experience and his suffering—went hand in hand. The fact that I shared in it with him allowed for empathy and sympathy.

Suffering is everywhere, yes. Yet, if you zoom far enough out to consider the world on a global scale, the terrible things are vastly outnumbered by the good things. Cruelty is less common than kindness, destruction can't keep up with creative energy and ingenuity, and even the worst atrocities stand out as horrific exceptions to the general rule.

We also tend to notice negative things more than positive things. There's a term for that in psychology: "negativity bias." It's one of many cognitive biases that cause us to misunderstand the world around us. Bad news makes for more exciting headlines, and those get more clicks. Bad news also tends to happen more quickly than good news. It's easier and quicker to destroy something than to build it—so the pace of new bad news is faster. That's why it seems like there's more bad than good.

Consider traffic lights. When we're driving a car and trying to get somewhere, it seems like we hit nothing but red lights. But that's not true. It's just that we tend to remember the red lights—the green lights escape our memory. We don't remember as much when things are going smoothly.

Of course, negative stuff does happen. Suffering—the pain of experience—is part of the deal when it comes to mattering, to having personal significance. If we never suffered, we wouldn't get a chance to matter.

There's a reason suffering tends to bring us together.

Sometimes, joy and suffering are intertwined. Sometimes they go hand in hand. If we aim for a path free of suffering, we're going to be disappointed. It's part of the journey. Acknowledging and accepting that early on can help set you up to endure the challenges ahead. If you're familiar at all with Buddhism, you might know that the first of the Four Noble Truths is that life is full of suffering. There's a reason why this truth comes first—because we need to accept it up front. It's part of the deal when it comes to being human. It's also why we learn early on, in the earliest books of the Old Testament, about the cause of what we call "original sin" in Christianity. The mess is wired in. You might say it's a feature, not a bug—or, at least, it's the original bug, and it's been part of us long enough to have become a feature.

When I was a younger teacher, I used to tell students going through a difficult patch that "everything was going to be okay." Now, as a middle-aged guy, I acknowledge that was bad advice—well intentioned, but nonetheless bad advice. Truth is, *not* everything is going to be okay in your life. In fact, unless you lead a truly fortunate existence, some parts of your life are probably going to be terrible. The important thing to remember, though, is that (at least for most people), most of life isn't terrible, most of the time.

Another thing to consider about suffering is that if we didn't suffer, we wouldn't know its opposite. You can't have light without darkness, sweet without bitter, smooth without rough. Our suffering is part of what allows us to be human together. I know it seems strange, but think of how life would be if there were *no* suffering involved. Take a few minutes to think about it: If there were no suffering, then what would you strive for? What would motivate you? In fact, why would anyone do *anything* at all? I'm not being trite or trying to glorify suffering. I'm just making the point: suffering is at the core of the human experience.

Men of the Earth

Father David Fleming, SJ, explained in one of his books that the word "human" comes from the Latin word *humus*, which means "earth."[1] So, to be human is to be "of the earth." The more you think about it, the more it makes sense.

The same linguistic origins are shared by "humble," "humility," and "humiliation." We say a wise man is "well grounded" and "has both feet on the ground." When we fail, we speak of downfalls, being laid low, or knocked flat. Creation stories suggest our mortal bodies are formed from clay. When our mortal bodies expire, we bury them in the earth or reduce them to ash and dust.

In the meantime, we're all a beautiful mess. Imperfect. Humble. This goes for everyone. Guys. Girls. Whatever ethnicity. Whatever nationality. Whatever color, language, or accent. Whatever sexuality. Whatever religion, or no religion. Everyone. We're all imperfect, and we all create our own beautiful little human mess.

You, Sam, and I are just men of the earth.

Sam and I have remained close over the years. He's had a rough path. But he knows that he matters, and he keeps striving, well aware of his own messiness. I encourage him, and he encourages me. We often talk about our respective messes. We talk about the things we suffer, our *pathos*, just as much as we talk about life's joys.

And in the meantime, we both strive for *arete*. We both know that getting there requires virtue—making a habit of doing the right thing—and that's a journey in itself.

So, let's talk about virtue.

CHAPTER THREE

Getting to Virtue

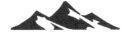

SPEEDING TICKETS. Man, I used to get a lot of them. Six before age twenty-two—about once a year. Funny thing is, I got at least two of them, maybe even three, at the exact same speed trap on a highway outside of Buffalo that I traveled frequently.

You'd think I'd learn better, right?

Except, if you ask people if they're good drivers, almost everyone will say yes. An old bit of wisdom in the insurance industry is that 80 percent of drivers think they're better than average, and psychological studies suggest the same thing.[1] Obviously, 80 percent of people can't be better than average. Do the math.

What about you? Do you consider yourself a good driver? If you'd asked me when I was twenty, I would have insisted that I was a better driver than most people. And yet I got all those speeding tickets and I had a couple fender benders, too. It wasn't until I'd accumulated a collection of speeding tickets that I realized I hadn't really been a good driver at all. The proof was right there.

The American historian Will Durant famously (and excellently, I think) rephrased some wisdom from the Greek philosopher Aristotle, putting it like this: "We are what we repeatedly do. Excellence, then, is not an act, but a habit."[2] Durant paraphrased some of the oldest wisdom in the world, and we can learn a lot from old wisdom.

What Is Virtue?

Aristotle's *Nicomachean Ethics* invites us to consider the best manner of living.[3] In it, Aristotle suggests that virtues are the characteristics of a person who aims his actions toward what is good by avoiding extremes. For example, the virtue of courage is between recklessness and cowardice; likewise, there's a healthy level of virtuous ambition that lies between too little, which would be laziness, and too much, which would be dangerous. Furthermore, Aristotle tells us that becoming a person of virtue depends on making a *habit* of doing the right thing. Aristotle goes into quite a bit of depth on this and it gets fairly complicated, but I think a good starting place to understand virtue is to focus on this idea of doing the right thing as a matter of habit. In other words, working hard to make it our "default setting."

But to make doing the right thing our default setting is no easy prospect. To be fair, doing the right thing *some* of the time is not that hard. But doing the right thing habitually? Consistently? Even when no one is watching? That's much harder. If we have to make virtuous behavior a habit in order to become virtuous men, well, that means we have to work at it. In other words, virtue takes practice—developing good habits takes time. In fact, I think we have to go through stages of habit-building before we really get good at virtues.

To explain what I mean, I'll ask you to consider an example focused on driving. Let's assume that driving responsibly reflects the virtue of personal responsibility. If we want to be truly responsible drivers, we have to drive conscientiously on a repeated, consistent basis—not just when there's a police officer nearby or when the weather is particularly bad. So, let's imagine four different drivers at different stages of developing the virtue of responsibility in their driving habits. Specifically, let's consider their habits around speeding.

The first guy doesn't obey the rules at all. He might be ignorant, careless, or willfully disobedient. He doesn't have much regard for his own safety or that of others. Even the threat of a speeding ticket isn't enough to keep him in line. Not only has he not habituated good driving habits; he's actually habituated bad ones. He's about as far from the virtue of responsibility as you can get, and it's probably going to take some time and experience before he builds good habits. Hopefully no one will get hurt in the meantime.

Our next guy isn't totally reckless. To be sure, he's not thinking too much about safety. But he knows that if he speeds, he might get pulled over, get a ticket, have points applied to his license, and get in serious trouble with his parents. He sticks to the speed limit because he *fears consequences*. He's obedient. The rules of the road are playing an important role in helping him develop responsible habits. His default setting is not necessarily to drive responsibly, but fear of consequences presses him to move in that direction—as much as he might not like it.

Our third driver has had a few speeding tickets, so he's aware of the consequences. But that's not the only reason he drives responsibly. After a while, he's realized that rules of the road are *useful*. Sure, he'd maybe prefer to go faster, but he's learned it's better and less stressful for everyone—himself included—when people obey some simple rules. He gets aggravated when other people don't follow them. This third driver is *compliant*. He obeys the speed limit because he respects the *utility* of traffic laws as part of the whole transit system. His belief in the *usefulness* of the rules overpowers his impulse to speed. He is becoming more responsible. His default setting is closer to true responsibility.

Our last driver sticks to the speed limit and follows other rules because he knows it's the right thing to do. Sure, maybe he's gotten speeding tickets, but he's learned from those experiences. Yes, he's realized that the entire highway traffic system just works better when people stick to the rules. But it goes beyond that for him. He obeys the law because he genuinely desires the good. He obeys the law to best ensure the safety of himself, his passengers, and others on the road—but even *that* isn't enough. He obeys the law because he finds happiness, joy, and satisfaction in being a driver who does the right thing for its own sake. Responsible driving habits have become his default setting.

This last guy, I think Aristotle would suggest, is the most virtuous driver. Doing the right thing has truly become a habit for him. Does this mean that if we aren't doing good things *exclusively* for the sake of the moral good itself, that we aren't virtuous? I don't think it's quite that simple. If our motivation is like the second or third drivers—that is, either obedience out of fear or compliance rooted in respect for what's practical—we are certainly more virtuous than that first idiot—the guy who doesn't care at all. At the same time, though, we aren't *as* virtuous as the guy who does the right thing just to do the right thing. We're on the way to refining our default settings. Our habits are becoming more virtuous; hence, our virtues are becoming more habituated.

So, if you're like driver number one, do us all a favor and get off the road. Chances are, though, you're more like driver two or three. That's good! That's a moral development as you make your path. Maybe you're more like driver four. I'd like to think I am—but not because I'm a paragon of virtue. It's at least in part simply because I'm a middle-aged dad driving a minivan full of kids. Sometimes our responsibilities shape our virtues. But the important point here is that you don't have to be a middle-aged dad driving a minivan to be a virtuous driver. You just have to develop a *habit* of driving conscientiously.

The Power of Habit

"We are what we repeatedly do."

By the time you're old enough to read a book like this, you are old enough to understand this and know it from your own experience.

We are creatures of habit. There are neurological reasons for this. Our brains get better at doing what we repeatedly do. Scientists know that due to neuroplasticity, our brain actually rewires itself—literally—in response to our repeated habits. This explains "muscle memory" and how we master things like riding a bike or typing without looking at the keyboard.

Consider even the most trivial, everyday routines. Think about the way you brush your teeth. You probably follow the same pattern of movements with your toothbrush each time. You might think it seems random, but it probably isn't. When you step out of the shower and reach for the towel, how do you dry yourself off? Think it's random and different each time? Probably not. I bet you follow the same pattern of movements.

Our habits build patterns, and our patterns reinforce our habits. It's a self-perpetuating cycle. "We are what we repeatedly do." The tricky thing is, we are good at seeing patterns in other people's behavior, but not in our own. When my parents saw my pattern of speeding tickets, they knew I wasn't being a careful driver. But I didn't see it that way. I saw each one as a special circumstance or an exception to my general driving habits.

If you want a better understanding of yourself, you have to get better at recognizing your *patterns*. That takes attention, honesty, and humility. Attention to see them in the first place, honesty to acknowledge the truth about what you do, and humility to understand that you're a creature of habit just like everyone else. Consider a few examples.

It doesn't make much sense to claim to be an organized person and yet be constantly disorganized. Do you know that guy? It doesn't make much sense to claim to be a dedicated athlete and teammate and yet repeatedly skip workouts. Know him? What about that guy who wouldn't call himself a screen addict but compulsively checks his phone hundreds of times each day? What about the guy who thinks of himself as healthy but eats junk food almost every day? What about the guy who considers himself honest but has a regular habit of cheating on minor homework assignments? What about the guy who would never consider himself hooked on internet porn but in fact watches it—hey, just for a few minutes—almost every night?

Of course, this can be more serious, too. Talk to someone who has accepted the truth that he's an alcoholic, and he'll probably tell you that he didn't see his patterns of addiction until someone or something forced him to.

Habit is really powerful. We are what we repeatedly do. Negative habits reinforce themselves. Positive habits reinforce themselves. That means we build our own patterns. We can also change them, but that takes work—and, usually, some rules.

Why We Need Rules

We need rules because "we are what we repeatedly do." Habits don't form in an instant. They form over time. If we want to build good patterns, and avoid building bad ones, we need some rules in place. These help us build a sort of moral muscle memory.

Think of the simple rules we teach little kids in kindergarten, for example. They're some of the most important rules we have. They form the basic patterns of common decency. They are very clear, simple, and consistent. Always do this; never do that. Think of the mantra you repeat during driver education courses: Buckle up. Adjust your mirrors. Check your gauges. Both hands on the steering wheel. Check your blind spot. These rules become habits. Consider your family. What rules are imposed to form good habits and avoid bad ones? Would you form different habits if those rules weren't there?

Maybe you're an athlete. What rules does your team have? What would happen if those rules were just suggestions? Ever try to get stronger and set up a workout plan for yourself? You'll probably see a big difference in results if you consider following your routine a rule instead of a suggestion.

The beauty of Aristotle's ancient wisdom—and the sophisticated science of neuroplasticity that we now understand—is that as we build good habits, we depend less on the rules that shaped them. And as we build good habits, we become more virtuous. We need rules to *form* habits, which can then become virtues. Little by little.

GETTING STRONGER, LITTLE BY LITTLE

Strength is really important. Physical strength matters for sure, but you know there are many kinds of strength. One of the most important is the strength of personal discipline, and we achieve that little by little. Let me tell you a cool story about this slow, steady kind of progress.

My dad retired several years ago from a five-decade career as a primary care physician and infectious disease specialist. By the time he closed up shop and hung up his stethoscope in his late seventies, he'd taken care of thousands of patients.

He was able to join me at a speaking engagement at a boys' boarding school. It was a two-day workshop focused on healthy masculinity. I've done a handful of these consulting gigs over the past several years, and I thought it would be fun to have my dad along for one. I figured he'd have plenty to offer, having raised five sons and with all his years in medicine. I was right. He brought a lot to it.

One moment stands out. We were talking to a group of teachers who lived with the guys in the dorms. I had been talking about the path to virtue—I used the speed limit example—and how important it is to encourage boys as they try to become more virtuous, even if it's only little by little. My dad, prompted by this, stepped in and offered a memorable story.

Several years ago, he was working with a very overweight patient. This patient asked him how he stayed so lean. Dad explained that he ran every day.

The patient scoffed. "Look at me! How could I run?"

Dad smiled and told him to walk instead.

"I can't even walk to the end of the block!" the man exclaimed. "I get so out of breath."

Dad asked him if he could walk around the dining room table. "Of course," he replied. "But what good would *that* do?"

Dad told him to begin walking around the dining room table, just three times a day for a week. He did.

He called the office a week later. "I did it. I walked around the table three times every day this week. In fact, yesterday, I did it four times."

Dad encouraged him and upped the dosage to ten laps of the dining room table, twice a day, for two weeks. The next time the man called, he was disappointed, because he'd missed a day. My dad encouraged him. He said it was a lapse, but that we needed to get over our lapses and press on. So, the man did it. He was excited when he called again.

"Doc, I doubled what you said! I started at ten laps, but now I've been doing twenty laps a day for a whole week!"

This went on for a while. Eventually, Dad challenged the man to walk to the corner and back—with his daughter along to help him. He did it.

Soon, he was taking walks *around* the block. Within a few months, he'd lost enough weight that it began to show, and he began to feel better. A year and a half later, the man had lost more than a hundred pounds. He never did become a runner, but he became a walker, and with that improved level of fitness, he also became a much happier man.

He needed to start with a simple rule to govern his behavior until the behavior became a habit. But none of this, my dad explained, would have happened if the man were too prideful or pessimistic to see the value of a single lap around the dining room table.

You can get stronger, but it's often—usually, in fact—little by little.

VIRTUE IS HARD, SO BE CAREFUL WITH JUDGMENT

A final thought on virtue: be careful with judgment.

It's true that building good habits takes discipline. You have to hold yourself to standards and follow rules if you want them to become good habits. But be careful to understand the difference between accountability and judgment.

Accountability means holding yourself—or someone else—to a standard or expectation, and being honest when and if it isn't met. Usually, this leaves room for improvement. It's kind of like saying to someone, "Because I believe in you and I know you can do better, I'm going to call you out on this, so you can change." That's encouraging. Hopefully, you've been held accountable by people who love you. It's what we mean when we say "tough love."

Judgment, on the other hand, goes a step further and leads to a *conclusion* about a person because of a failure. It has a kind of finality about it. It isn't encouraging. In fact, it sort of slams the door on the possibility of change. It's like saying, "What you did is enough to define you in my eyes, and there's no point in my looking any further."

On a larger scale, we see this in the "cancel culture" and "calling out" that plays out in social media mobs. But I think we see it often in small ways, too, in our own circle of family and friends, where it probably means more. Has this happened among your family and friends? Have you felt the sort of lasting grudge that such judgment imposes on a relationship? It isn't pretty.

It isn't hard to become judgmental. To be fair, sometimes judgment is justly earned. People can be pretty lousy, and the expression "you reap what you sow" has real meaning. But I think we should be very careful about coming to judgmental conclusions about people. You could say that Aristotle's wisdom (as rephrased by Durant) that "we are what we repeatedly do" is a sort of judgment. Fair point, but it also implies that we can always change. It isn't "we are what we repeatedly *did*." It's "we are what we repeatedly *do*."

I hate to go all English teacher on you, but the verb tense *really* matters here. No one wants to be judged solely on his worst moment or greatest failure, as though there's no possibility of redemption, right? I sure don't. Do you?

It's Supposed to Be Hard!

The quest for the moral excellence embodied in virtue is difficult indeed. It takes self-discipline to follow the rules that build good habits. Would you expect something so important to be easy? And yet the challenge makes the quest aspirational. It's hopeful. It's encouraging, even as it is difficult. As long as we are breathing, and if we intend to make our path climb higher, there remains the possibility of attaining moral virtue, despite our failings. We should be patient with ourselves and others as we make our paths.

Climbing is slow, difficult work.

Our path is made of our experiences, and they take a while to accumulate. I'll leave with a final quick story about how I finally became a good driver.

I became an emergency medical technician (EMT) in my early twenties. I only did this for a few years, as a volunteer with a small fire department, but I learned a lot on those calls. Occasionally, I had to drive an ambulance pretty fast. Each time, my heart pounded and adrenaline pumped as the lights flashed and siren blared.

Seeing what can happen when people get hurt on the road gave me a new appreciation of seatbelts, speed limits, and traffic lights. I gained a newfound respect for the rules. This changed my habits.

If you'd called me a reckless driver at nineteen, I would have argued with you. But my speeding tickets would have been all the proof you needed. More than twenty-five years later, I can say with confidence that I'm *actually* a good driver, and part of the proof is that I haven't had a speeding ticket in many years.

Fair to say we *were* what we repeatedly *did*.

But . . .

We *are* what we repeatedly *do*.

CHAPTER FOUR

Failure and Regret

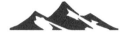

SWEAT POURED DOWN THE SIDES of my sunburned face. I was doubled over, hands on my knees, trying desperately to catch my breath after sprinting to the finish of the obstacle course. My T-shirt, completely soaked, clung to my body. Fellow cadets clapped me on the back as the drill instructor called out my elapsed time from the stopwatch.

It was July 1997. I was eighteen and somewhere in the first or second week of Swab Summer at the US Coast Guard Academy in New London, Connecticut. The air was sultry as I, along with the rest of my cadet platoon, wrapped up a tough morning on the obstacle course.

Later that night, after a day that had already seemed to last seventy-two hours, I stood at attention in the corridor of Chase Hall with the rest of my company, going through repeated rifle drills, sets of pushups, and recitations of memorized bits of knowledge called "rates." When asked, for example, "Cadet, what's your piece?" the response was, "Sir, my piece is US Rifle, M-1, Caliber .30, gas operated, clip-fed, air-cooled, semiautomatic shoulder weapon, sir!"

At the end of the drill period, I was surprised to hear my name called. My heart raced as I stepped forward, executed a sharp ninety-degree turn, and paced to the older cadet in charge of our platoon. I stood trembling, shoulders back and chest out, bracing for the worst. It could have been about anything—an improperly made rack, something out of place on my uniform, or a lapse in how I had handled my rifle.

Instead, I was recognized for leadership and impressive performance under pressure. I was named platoon "guidon" (pronounced "guide-on"). It was a minor leadership post that would last just a couple of days before being turned over to another cadet, but it was a notable honor. I would call out cadences and carry our platoon's flag. Later that night, after we'd showered and enjoyed the five minutes of nightly down time before *Taps* would call for us to hit the rack, my peers congratulated me. There were high-fives, fist-bumps, and good-natured words of affirmation.

As I lay in my rack that night, my US Rifle, M-1, Caliber .30, gas-operated, clip-fed, air-cooled, semiautomatic shoulder weapon at my side, I felt very much a part of something. I felt pride. After eighteen years of hard work and discipline, I'd made it. I smiled as I thought of my dad, who'd served as a major in the Air Force during Vietnam. I thought of my two grandfathers. My dad was only fifteen when his father died, so I'd never met that grandfather. He was a staff sergeant in the

Army and served in both the Atlantic and Pacific theaters in World War II. My mom's father, who had always been one of my heroes, was a Navy veteran—and had been immensely proud of my decision to serve.

But like the tower in that story I told you in the beginning of this book, my aspirations in the Coast Guard proved unsteady, and my military career soon came crashing down. The aftermath nearly crushed me.

This is a chapter about failure and regret. More importantly, it's about how to handle them both so that you don't spend your life lost in the past. You don't know what the future holds, and you can't rewrite the past. In fact, the only time we get to do anything is in the present. And that's good, because we are what we repeatedly *do*.

BUILDING MY TOWER, AND SEEING IT FALL

I'd aspired to a military career since midway through high school. I loved everything nautical and had been scuba diving since age twelve. The Coast Guard especially drew me because of its humanitarian missions like search and rescue.

Gaining admission to any of the service academies like West Point, Annapolis, Air Force, or the Coast Guard Academy is very competitive, so when I was accepted to the Coast Guard Academy, my plans accelerated and the excitement grew. Everyone was proud. I was, I believed, living my dream.

But it didn't last.

Instead, I washed out of the Academy just weeks after that hot day on the obstacle course. I didn't even stay long enough to participate in one of the most storied traditions at the Academy, an extended training cruise on the tall ship *Eagle*. More than twenty-five years later, I'm still amazed at how quickly I quit.

For years, my ego and my shame teamed up and conspired to keep me from acknowledging that. I used to say things like "I decided to transfer," "I withdrew voluntarily," or "I felt called to become a teacher, instead." Those all sound better. And, of course, they're all true. But none of those lines tells the *whole* story. With enough distance and time, I finally took ownership of the truth, and I found that I could just admit it with two simple, clear words: I quit.

Things at the Academy had been okay at first—more than okay, actually. Along with being named guidon, I excelled in some of the core strength exercises. I was exceptional in the pool training after years of swimming and diving. I didn't mind the complete absence of privacy. Desensitized to the anxieties of being in close proximity with naked dudes by years on my high school crew team, I wasn't even fazed by the indignities of the "navy showers," which were very crowded and *very* short. We got about thirty seconds to wet down, shampoo, and rinse off, taking turns under the showerheads.

And like that night I was called forward before my platoon, there were other moments amid the hustle and rush and yelling and pushups and interminable sweating, when everything seemed to freeze in time, and I felt the joy of being a part of something bigger than myself. For example, there was one occasion when we assembled outside at night. I don't remember the details, but I think it must have been a recognition ceremony of some kind for a senior cadet, and there was some kind of patriotic music. What I do remember clearly is the stars and stripes snapping in a steady night breeze, the flag lit up by a spotlight, and a feeling of immense pride during our salute.

But I recall another very distinct memory. It was the middle of the night, a few weeks in. Our blinds must have been open because I remember moonlight on the wall. I was lying in my rack, with my rifle, of course. I was staring up at the glowing red indicator light on the smoke detector.

The thought hit me, hard: *Go home. This isn't right for you.*

I don't know why. I just had the strongest impulse to leave. It wasn't a familiar feeling. I'd never really quit anything up to that point. To quit would be to fail. I felt it in my gut. But I did it anyway. Just a few days later, despite long, meaningful, serious urgings from my cadre cadets and the Academy chaplain, I signed my withdrawal papers and shipped home.

On that final day, I'd awoken to the trumpeted tones of *Reveille* in the barracks and donned the uniform of my country, a remarkable education and career before me. By the time I fell asleep that night, I was back in my childhood bed, staring up at the glow-in-the-dark stars I'd stuck to the ceiling when I was nine.

Many years later, I now understand that at age eighteen, I made a major life decision aimed at becoming the *idea* of something rather than becoming the actual thing itself. I'd been aiming to build a tower, when my vocation was, in fact, to be a bridge-builder. Problem was, I didn't know it.

My Experience of Depression

Coming back to Buffalo was terrible for a lot of reasons. Down came the posters and the ship's wheel and the maritime knick-knacks that had adorned my bedroom throughout high school. I sure as hell didn't want anything to do with boats or ships. In a fit of now-hilarious melodrama, I smashed my CD with the *Top Gun* soundtrack and threw out my previously beloved military movie collection of VHS tapes.

I did not enjoy seeing *Titanic* when it came out later that winter.

If you hadn't heard, the damn ship sinks.

The local Jesuit college honored the scholarship it had offered. I enrolled there as an English major, falling back on my known strengths. But then I started spending a lot of evenings alone, staring at those stars on the ceiling. The thing about depression, which I think a lot of people misunderstand, is that it isn't a lot of weeping and sadness. Oh, sure, I did enough weeping. Eventually, though, that stopped. In its more advanced form, depression isn't *feeling* anything. It's the opposite—it's numbness. It's kind of like hypothermia. We shiver when it's setting in, for sure. But you know it's getting really serious when the shivering *stops*.

I was stuck in the past, so I was paralyzed in the present.

I spiraled pretty quickly over the next year and a half into an outright clinical depression. A lot of people tried to help me, and a few pharmaceutical suggestions were offered by well-meaning doctors, including my father and brother. I rejected them all.

This was my biggest mistake in this entire situation: trying so damned hard to go it alone. When you're going through depression, it's hard to ask for help. Part of what makes it so hard is that it's difficult to articulate what you're feeling—or not feeling. How do you tell someone what's wrong when you don't know what's wrong? I remember longing to be able to share what I was feeling (or not feeling), but not knowing how to describe it. The very thought of trying to describe what depression feels like—actually, make that *doesn't* feel like—is exhausting.

So yeah. I spent a couple years exhausted. Empty tank. Coasting in neutral. I became addicted to my own misery. When you feel paralyzed and numb, sometimes you go for the most accessible thing there is just to remind yourself that you're not totally numb: pain.

Pain as a remedy?

Yep. If that sounds twisted, it's because it is.

Depression is a twisted snake feeding on its own tail.

After all these years, I no longer regret leaving the Academy, but I regret pushing everyone away and my stubborn refusal to accept help. I regret the relationships with close high school friends that I damaged in the aftermath. I regret the turmoil and worry I inflicted on my parents, extended family, friends, and mentors. Mostly, I regret the stubborn insistence on handling it by myself, even though I clearly couldn't.

If any of this sounds familiar to you, let me tell you, based on personal experience: swallow your pride and ask for help! If you ask—if you can muster the humility to truly seek it out—it will be there. It might be in unexpected places, and it might take a while to find, but it is there.

In an attempt to help them avoid my mistake, I've encouraged many boys and young men to get professional counseling and therapy over the years. I have a firm belief in the transformative power of getting help, whether it is medication, counseling, or something like cognitive behavioral therapy, which aims to help people more clearly understand and cope with their struggles. It helps them climb out.

RECOVERY: CLIMBING OUT

So, if I didn't seek help the way I should have, what freed me from this paralysis of living in the past? The love of my parents, family, friends, and mentors. That was the fundamental precondition for my recovery. Relationships help us climb out of the dark. We don't do it alone. Can you think of relationships that have helped you at the lowest parts of your life?

Of course, it isn't just people. Sometimes events can change everything, too. Sometimes the present moment is so powerful—so life-altering—that it jolts us out of the past for good.

For me, that moment was September 11, 2001.

I graduated from college in 2001, and I knew by then that I wanted to teach at a Jesuit high school. The Jesuits had played a big role in my life, and my spirituality had deepened quite a bit during college. (More on that later.) After a rigorous set of interviews, I was honored to accept a position at Georgetown Prep in Bethesda, Maryland. My position there entailed three major roles: assistant chaplain, English teacher, and residential prefect.

As assistant chaplain, I ran much of the retreat program, helped with chapel duties, and trained the senior peer-mentors known as "Big Brothers." The actual chaplain was a Jesuit priest; as his assistant, part of my job was to serve as a sort of "backup" spiritual advisor to the kids—being someone younger and *not* a priest. As a prefect, I lived in the dorms and supervised residential life. I taught ninth-grade religion and English.

Shortly before class on 9/11, I was in my office and began to see the headlines about American Airlines Flight 11. I headed up toward the admin wing to be sure the chaplain and the other administrators knew what had happened. As I was passing the library, I saw a small crowd of teachers and students gathered around a television. During the time between leaving my office and then, the second tower had been hit.

Suddenly, everything changed. I gathered in the headmaster's office in a huddle with the rest of the administrative team, each of us trying to wrap our heads around the situation.

It was during that meeting that President Bush issued his statement announcing what had happened. It was also during that meeting that the Pentagon, just eleven miles away, was hit. We learned that the aunt of one of our students was a flight attendant on one of the planes.

My heart was pounding. We watched the South Tower disintegrate on live television. By that point, the roar of fighter jets overhead became a frequent sound, as did sirens.

Before our meeting ended, the chaplain told me that he needed to attend to the student who'd lost his aunt. I would be the chaplain on duty for the boarding students. He wanted me to gather them in the chapel that evening for a prayer service. "What should I do?" I remember asking. "Go with your gut," he replied. "You got this."

That evening, after dinner, we gathered in the darkened chapel. I offered a few words.

I encouraged them to lean on each other amid the fear.

I reminded them to love one another.

I challenged them not to be consumed by anger.

We passed a candle from person to person, and each guy had a chance to offer a prayer. As I looked up at the earnest faces in that room, many wet with tears illuminated by the candles, I felt what I now know to call "consolation." It was a profound sense of affirmation and purpose.

It wasn't happiness; far from it. It wasn't a feeling of success. It was the conviction that I was exactly where I was supposed to be, doing exactly what I was supposed to be doing. As though everything I'd struggled through over the past four years—the uncertainty, the confusion, the regret, the shame—disintegrated in that chapel.

That moment of super-clarity occurred at roughly the mid-point of my life to date. Since then, comparably much bigger things have happened, namely marriage and fatherhood. Yet, at the time, as a single guy, having struggled through the toughest years I'd had, it was everything to me.

I realized my decision to leave the Academy—to quit—didn't have to define my life. It was a difficult decision, and it wasn't without cost. But I found that I no longer regretted it.

USEFUL REGRETS VERSUS REGRETS THAT TRAP US

I've also made some genuinely *bad* decisions in my life. Some real failures. And yes, I do regret them.

I bet you do, too. Can you think of some?

There is a place for regret inside us, a part of the mechanism of memory that keeps us from repeating our mistakes and inflicting more pain than is necessary upon ourselves and others. That's useful, because it helps us be our best self in the present.

Of the regrets you thought of, which ones are this kind of "useful"?

Other regrets keep us living in the past, obsessing over failures we can't change and second-guessing ourselves. Those regrets aren't useful. They cloud our vision by trapping us in the past. They interfere with our ability to live in the present.

Again, consider your regrets. Are there any like this, that keep you trapped? Let go of those. Because the only time we get to do anything is in the present.

What does a focus on the present mean? *How* do you live in the present? Well, it's simple—but not necessarily easy. It means making an effort to be grateful for the people and opportunities that surround you at any given moment, *right now*. It means trying to notice, appreciate, and act on the possibilities that lie around you, *right now*.

A trick I use to help me live in the present is to always stay aware that what is now the present will soon be in the past—and once it is, I won't be able to change it. So, since I want to be able to look back on it without regrets, I have to invest myself in it while I have the chance. That might sound crazy, but it helps! Live your present moment so that it becomes a past moment you can look back on with satisfaction—or even a healthy level of pride.

Will it always work?

Nope. Sometimes it won't work, and you'll still live your present moment in a way that will generate regret. But a lot of the time, it will work, if you remain conscious that the current present moment will soon become part of your past.

Leaving the Academy turned out to be a good decision that took a long time to understand. I used to regret it; I don't anymore. The kid sweating on the obstacle course on that hot July day in 1997 was full of good intentions, but he was confused. He thought he was supposed to build a tower. He had an idea about who and what he wanted to be. Well, the tower of my original dream may have fallen, but my career has been full of bridge-building, starting on the day those Twin Towers fell.

When I see my wife and kids and think about the life we've built together, what can I possibly regret? Maybe that's a key indicator: if a regret fades over time, it means you've moved on. If it doesn't, you're letting yourself stay trapped by it.

Allowing regret to consume your life is like walking backwards, with your eyes focused uselessly on the ground you've already traveled. That's a hell of a tripping hazard.

I'm going to say it again, because it's so important:

The only time we get to do anything is in the present.

While these events on 9/11 solidified that realization, I have to take you back a little further—a year earlier, on the other side of the world—to explain the awakening that led to it.

Chapter Five

Life as Pilgrimage

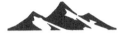

At six o'clock in the morning on Saturday, August 12, 2000, I woke up early to the sound of festival drums. After just a couple weeks in Nepal, I'd learned that every day was a festival.

And that these festivals involved drumming.

Often, a lot of drumming.

At all hours.

Stretching, I climbed from my tiny bunk in the shelter of a tiny trekking outpost located at high altitude in the Langtang region of the Himalayas. Sore and stinky from the rigorous climb that brought us there, I grumbled as I made my way, clad in thermal underwear and a fleece jacket, toward the tiny kitchen to drink some tea. I was dehydrated and far from acclimated to the high altitude.

That's when I spotted a rare sight—a sunbeam. Excited, I grabbed my camera; threw on my hat, socks, and boots; and went outside.

It was monsoon season. That meant nearly constant overcast, rainy weather. And that, of course, meant rarely catching a glimpse of the immense Himalayan peaks around us.

The clouds broke as the sun climbed higher, and I saw the Ganesh Himal in its glory. Suddenly, the world was different. It took on an enormity and a majesty that I had never imagined possible, especially in that dark time of my life.

That sunrise brought me to tears. It was a remarkable gift. It is one of those distinct moments, like the one I would have a year later on 9/11, that radically altered the trajectory of my life. That singular moment was part of what I now understand is my lifelong pilgrimage—a physical and spiritual journey that has continued ever since.

What Is Pilgrimage?

When most Americans hear the word "pilgrim," they probably think of Thanksgiving and the stories of the settlers who sailed to North America on the *Mayflower*, seeking freedom from religious persecution. Pilgrimage is a global phenomenon, though, and an ancient tradition that appears in cultures all over the world. Any transformative journey could be considered a pilgrimage and the person undertaking it a pilgrim. I like the way that Phil Cousineau, an author and documentary screenwriter, explains it:

> *By definition any journey is physically difficult, but pilgrimage is also spiritually challenging. It demands that we follow*

our spiritual compass and put the soles of our shoes to the soul of the world. It means getting back in touch with our earth, our roots, ourselves.[1]

A pilgrimage, then, is a challenging journey that deepens our understanding of ourselves and the world around us. It transforms us and makes us more fully human.

I think all of life is a pilgrimage, and I challenge you to look at your own life as one.

Where has your path taken you?

How has that journey deepened your understanding of yourself and the world around you?

How has it transformed you and made you fully human?

When you start to look at your life as a pilgrimage, you gain a new appreciation for the experiences that have formed your path. You also gain a new level of excitement, because you realize just how much possibility lies ahead!

JOURNEY TO THE REALM OF SNOW

Just a year before the events of 9/11 that I told you about in the last chapter, I had an experience that cemented this idea of pilgrimage in my mind and heart.

My oldest brother, Tom, to whom this book is dedicated, led me to the other side of the world when I was twenty-one. Busy with his internal medicine residency at Johns Hopkins and deeply immersed in international epidemiology research, he nonetheless saw the depressed shape I was in and invited me to join him on the second of three research expeditions to Nepal. This small country, known best for being the home of Mt. Everest, is nestled in the heart of the world's tallest mountain range, the Himalayas, which means "realm of snow."

I was a good writer and I'd been developing an amateur photography business, so he gave me the important-sounding title of "expedition journalist." I was also flat broke, so he paid most of my way, including buying some of my trekking and photography gear.

Also joining us would be Tom's longtime friend, D.J. Radder, who is one of the most adaptable, friendly, and open-minded people I've ever met. They'd already been friends since childhood, and Tom knew that despite his lack of medical expertise, D.J. was the ideal travel companion. He's a jack of all trades—the kind of guy who can tie fancy knots, fix broken gear, splice wires, patch tents, and charm his way through just about any dicey situation.

He's like human duct tape. The kind of guy you want with you on the road.

Maybe you know someone like that. If you were headed to the other side of the world, who would you want at your side? It's worth thinking about for a moment.

Our destination was a high-altitude lake called Gosain-kunda. After getting organized in Kathmandu with the rest of the medical team from the Himalayan Rescue Association, we'd pack our gear onto an overcrowded bus into the mountains for a sixteen-hour climb on rugged roads, as far as it could take us.

From there, we'd trek on foot, climbing several thousand feet each day and acclimatizing to the altitude overnight.

Gosainkunda is a sacred body of water situated at 14,366 feet of altitude—about ten thousand feet higher than Kathmandu. Thousands of Nepali pilgrims ascend there annually for the festival of Janai Purnima. According to tradition, it was formed by the trident of the god Shiva, the patron of the Kathmandu valley. The pilgrimage involves ritual bathing in the waters for redemption, purification, and renewal, with the changing of sacred Janai threads worn around the wrists.

My brother's field research examined the relationship between dehydration and altitude-related illnesses. The crowded pilgrimage to Gosainkunda would provide a large sample set for plenty of data. It was also likely that there would be a need for medical care, since many of the pilgrims ascend rapidly in just one or two days, making the trip without sufficient stops to adjust to the altitude.

D.J. was charged with rigging up a field clinic. Many travelers would come from remote mountain villages that rarely saw a doctor, so they would likely be eager to visit with a medical team. They would have a chance to be examined by the doctors and the rest of the team, and receive basic treatment if needed. If they agreed to participate in the study, we would measure their blood pressure and blood oxygen saturation, collect urine samples, and conduct diagnostic surveys.

As the prospect of this challenging journey to the far side of the world began to dawn on me, I felt a kind of energy I hadn't felt since leaving the Academy. I was intrigued and excited. Looking back, I understand now that the experience represented the total opposite of the depression I was in. Where I felt numb, it offered a plentitude of sensation. Where I felt inertia, it was pure momentum—both across the globe by plane and up the mountains by foot. Where I felt a lack of purpose, it presented a demanding set of important tasks essential to meaningful research. Where I felt complacent, it compelled action. Where I felt alone, it immersed me in community. It forced my eyes, ears, and other senses to snap out of their sleep. The experience, the research project, the exposure to the gut-wrenching poverty of the developing world—indeed, the entire undertaking—compelled me to get over myself. It was an awakening.

Can you think of a time when you've been really stoked for an upcoming challenge? Something you knew would push you outside your comfort zone? That's part of what pilgrimage offers us—it's intimidating and energizing all at once. It keeps our senses sharp and our mind and heart open. Not a bad way to look at every day, right?

Pilgrimage Helps Us Understand Ourselves

A few nights before we began our expedition, I'd been up late at night at a seedy bar in Kathmandu. I'd sat sipping Kingfisher beer and chatting in broken English with a guy just a few years older—he'd been on the path to become a Buddhist monk but decided against it, served in the Nepali Army for a couple years, and now worked as a tour guide.

We traded philosophical banter for a while—mostly alcohol-fueled nonsense, I'm sure—but part of our conversation stays with me. Somewhere in the course of our conversation, when he was talking about his own failure to complete his training as a monk, he shared that he felt trapped by his own regret.

Sounded familiar to me.

I replied, "Maybe we just trap ourselves." He looked at me, smiled, and said, "My friend, you are right. We have to let go or the past will kill us." Shortly after that, we finished our beers and went our separate ways. I shuffled back through the humid, noisy, narrow streets of the Thamel tourist district to my hostel, cheekily named the "Hotel California."

Now, I have no idea who the guy was, and there's not a chance I'd ever be able to track him down, but his words kept echoing in my mind over the next few days as I climbed with the research team to the high-altitude shrine of Gosainkunda, where our medical study took place.

It was in that spectacular moment I told you about, watching that sunrise and spotting the Ganesh Himal, that I understood his words. It isn't because I was in the Himalayas. It wasn't even because the sunrise was beautiful. It was simply because for the first time since leaving the Academy, I began to let go. Not just so that I wouldn't be *trapped* in the past—I now understood the stakes were higher: It was "so the past wouldn't kill me."

But see, you don't have to go to the Himalayas to have a "sunrise moment" like that.

You don't even really need a sunrise.

Then again, it can help. And those are available daily.

Pilgrimage Helps Us See the World

Pilgrimage helps us see the world. It shows us new places, sure. But I mean something deeper. It helps us really *notice* the world around us. To become truly aware of it. To experience it in such a way that we genuinely think and learn about it. For example, during that journey I learned about Buddhism and Hinduism. I learned about the Eightfold Path toward Enlightenment, and I realized an ancient truth embodied in these traditions: that embracing life's suffering is a necessary part of being fully human.

We didn't just conduct a medical study. I became keenly aware of that suffering as my brother and the rest of our team treated maladies during those long days on the mountain. My basic first aid skills were rapidly tested and expanded. We assisted in the treatment of everything from cuts and burns to bacterial infections.

That so many pilgrim travelers persisted—despite knowing the dangers of rapid ascent to high altitude—was a testament to their faith. Many were elderly; few had shoes. The team had to carry one old man down to lower altitude on a stretcher in order to save his life. Tom diagnosed him with high-altitude pulmonary edema, which was filling his lungs with fluid. He made the choice stark: the man must descend immediately and rapidly or die on the mountain. The old man fought the decision. He wanted to complete the pilgrimage. Fortunately, his family convinced him to descend. He survived, but barely.

As the days passed, the crowd grew into the thousands in a gathering tent city. The weather deteriorated, bringing rain, wind, and snow. We began to hear reports of people who had died on the shores of the frigid lake. They'd persisted in their ascent despite worsening conditions and altitude-induced sicknesses. Their conviction to reach the lake was that strong.

We descended after several days. Life changed for me. The courage, persistence, suffering, and strength of the Nepali pilgrims showed me the rawness and fullness of life. That journey was a radical departure from everything familiar and comfortable. It shattered my conceptions of normalcy, broadened my knowledge of the wider world, and woke me up to the reality of global poverty.

I began to see the connection between other ancient traditions and my own Catholic tradition, and I saw that suffering and redemption were human universals. In particular, I finally understood why Saint Ignatius of Loyola, the founder of the Jesuit order that had educated me, was known as "the pilgrim saint."

It's worth noting that about a month into this trip, I got really sick. It was an adverse reaction to an antimalarial medication. It put me in a bad place, wreaking havoc not only on my gastrointestinal system but also seriously messing with my head. Because of it, I had to come home early. As aggravating as it was to have to leave, it didn't hit me with the weight of failure the way bailing out of the Academy did. Thinking back on it, I think the awakening I experienced on that journey enabled me to accept life's twists and turns in a different way. Leaving the Academy had left my soul tied up in knots. Coming home from the roof of the world was different. Sick as I was—and believe me, I was *sick*, man—I felt those interior knots loosening. I think some of them even came undone.

It was a turning point on my journey through Ignatian spirituality, which has been influential throughout my adult life. Maybe it's ironic that an immersion in a different religious tradition, in an environment so radically different from my own, was the very thing that helped me embrace my own religious tradition. Then again, the whole point of a pilgrimage is to be transformed and renewed by a challenging journey out of the familiar.

Pilgrimage Is Transformative

It was only upon my return to the United States—after my head cleared from the antimalarial meds—that I truly understood the journey as a pilgrimage. I found that it had sharpened my focus and helped me climb out of the doldrums of the previous three years. It rekindled my intellectual curiosity. I began to see the value of the bridge that I was building, despite the fallen tower of my failed military aspirations. That journey, and the people who accompanied me on it, transformed my understanding of life itself. I realized that each day is an opportunity to, as Cousineau wrote, "put the soles of our shoes to the soul of the world." From that time forward, I would consider all of life a pilgrim journey.

I still do.

EMBARK ON YOUR OWN PILGRIMAGE

Have you been on a challenging journey that deepened your understanding of yourself and the world around you? Pilgrimage can take many forms. There are literal physical journeys and metaphoric ones.

Metaphorically, a pilgrimage might be a challenging season with your team on the difficult road to a championship. It can be navigating a complicated relationship with someone you love. It could be working your way through a difficult course in high school, college, or trade school. It could be going through your teenage years with your parents and family, working your way through the tensions. It might be moving to a new city to take a job. No doubt you've been on some kind of pilgrimage like this in the course of everyday life. It takes many forms.

But one of the things I think is so important for boys and young men today is to embark on a "deep" pilgrimage experience. For all of human history, boys have undergone rites of passage to manhood. This is different in every culture, but it's a universal. While there are too many different rites of passage to begin describing here, you have no doubt heard of many. These rites of initiation mark a transition point from boyhood to manhood. The classical archetypal hero stories that fill our myths, legends, and folklore often portray boys and young men embarking on quests to gain the wisdom and experience needed to take on the burdens of manhood.

Contemporary society has diminished the intensity of these rites of passage, which is probably a good thing, especially considering some of them could be fatal. But perhaps our modern culture of convenience and technology has also cushioned things a little too much. Some risk—some danger—is good.

Without it, we don't get tested.

Without it, we're more likely to be paralyzed by fear.

Without it, we aren't sure how strong we are.

So I urge you to embark on some kind of communal quest that will engage you in rites of passage with others. Seek something full of challenges and trials that will require you to push yourself ahead, uphill. The most obvious way to do this is to join an athletic team. But it could also be an active club, or a youth group, or a volunteer service organization.

Go on a religious or meditative or wilderness retreat. Many such opportunities are out there. Most are mixed company, while some of them are just for women or just for men. While any such experience can be life changing, I suggest there may be value in seeking out something that's designed for just guys. For many men, all-male spaces foster a level of openness, transparency, and vulnerability that is elusive in mixed settings.

Most importantly, if you have the means, I challenge you to consider the possibility of a literal pilgrimage journey. This might be a trip you take with your school, your church, or some other organization. Maybe it will involve volunteer service (more on that later). It might be a road trip with family or friends. It might, in fact, be a multiday trek in the wilderness. Just make sure it's not an easy section of the path. If it's challenging enough, it *will* change you. It'll make you stronger. It'll make you less scared. It'll make you more patient. It'll make you kinder. It'll make you more fully human.

SEE YOUR LIFE AS A PILGRIMAGE

Like so many words in this book, pilgrimage finds its roots in Latin. It comes from *per agrum*, meaning "through the field." That implies it's not a straight path, like a paved road.

If you always travel on straight, paved roads, you're going to have an easier go of it. But there's a lot you're going to miss in this world. You have to step off the beaten path and make one of your own.

All of life is a pilgrimage, if you make it one.

Oh—and while you're out there, get up early enough to catch the sunrise.

Chapter Six

Learning as Adventure

Little kids love playgrounds. There's a special kind of delight on the faces of toddlers when they arrive at a playground on a bright summer morning. They scramble to undo their car seat buckles, hop down to the sidewalk, and run with all the speed their stubby little toddler legs can muster, squealing with joy. Within seconds they've scattered, already fully immersed in exploration, plunging among the various swings, slides, and ladders, running from one structure to another in a desperate rush to try everything out.

Playful Learning

Can you remember this? The start of a summer day, endless possibilities stretching ahead, with little thought of annoyances like eating vegetables, taking a bath, or brushing your teeth?

Do you remember the inventive, imagination-charged play you enjoyed? Games and contests that pitted your strength and will against imagined foes and evil villains? The imposing height of a slide, and the dizzy excitement of going just a little too high on the swings?

This kind of all-in, energetic play is analogous to real learning. The way little kids plunge headlong into the obstacle-riddled terrain of a playground bears many similarities to the way a genuinely curious mind probes the vast and varied landscape of ideas.

It's invigorating. Challenging. Rewarding. Sometimes, even dangerous. You can get hurt in the playground of the intellect. I once caught the edge of an imbalanced teeter-totter on the upswing with the center of my chin—and it was not a pleasant experience. This happened shortly after I succeeded in taking on the really big slide for the first time. There I was, still reveling in the glory of conquering that scary slide, even as blood poured from my mouth and my mom checked for missing teeth.

The playground can be dangerous, but that's where we learn what we can do, right? Where we push our limits and discover what we're made of. These are good things to do as we go about making our path. I'd like to propose that genuine learning can be just as exciting, challenging, dangerous, and rewarding as those summer days on the playground.

IS THE INTELLECTUAL PLAYGROUND CLOSED FOR BOYS AND MEN?

If you're like most young guys—at least in the United States—there's a good chance school doesn't feel much like an intellectual playground. For a lot of teenage boys and young men, school seems like the opposite of adventure. This can be pretty discouraging, and I think it's important to see how it's affecting this generation of young guys.

We can look at a few statistics that suggest something is going on in education, and it doesn't look great for boys and men. Consider reading, which is one of the most fundamental elements of education. First off, everyone knows that boys *on average* don't read as much as girls, which is probably as much temperamental as cultural. Second, academic achievement gaps are big, particularly in verbal areas, and boys aren't faring well. Richard Reeves (now president of the American Institute for Boys and Men) and Ember Smith authored a 2022 Brookings Institute research brief that puts this in stark terms, outlining a number of statistics. Among the most striking is the gap in reading achievement from grades four to eight: "Girls outperform boys in reading by more than 40 percent of a grade level in every state. In ten states . . . girls are more than a full grade level ahead of boys." The same document highlights the gap in on-time high school graduation rates, where the researchers estimated girls were ahead by 6.5 percentage points based on 2021 data.[1]

And then there's college enrollment. As the aforementioned Richard Reeves has rather famously pointed out, the gender gap has not only reversed; it has also widened. There was a 13 percent gender gap in college enrollment in 1972 in favor of men when the education bill Title IX was passed to try to address it. That gap has not only reversed, but it has also grown wider today than it was back then.[2] There are many more young women enrolled in college than young men. The latest data, which traces back to US enrollment in fall of 2021, indicates that for full-time undergraduate enrollment, it was 58 percent women and 42 percent men,[3] and the available projections suggest a similar gap will persist for the next decade.

In terms of who is actually *graduating* from college within six years (or, for that matter, at all), the percentage reflects a notable female majority. Considerably more women than men are entering both medical school and law school in the United States.

What about reading, beyond the context of education? Research from more than a decade ago showed most books are purchased, borrowed, and read by girls and women.[4] While more recent research from the Pew Research Center asserts that women are still more likely to read in general, it does suggest that when it comes to digital format books (e.g., ebooks and audiobooks), men and women are equally likely to read.[5] I find it interesting that these different media formats appear to be more appealing than print books to some men. Anecdotally, I know that listening to audiobook versions of the works I assign in class has benefited a good number of my male students. Some of them, who would probably not read print books voluntarily, have embraced audiobooks outside of school, too. This seems to be a positive development, but there's still work to do when it comes to encouraging boys and men to read.

Any one of these facts indicating an educational gap might not bear much significance on its own, but taken together, they clearly suggest boys and young men are trending *away* from the kind of intellectual pursuits at the heart of formal education—especially at the university level. What does this mean about the *kind* of thinking—the *depth* of thinking—men are doing? Boys and men make up half of the global population—are we spending enough time in the intellectual playground? Maybe not. I want boys and men to rediscover the joy of learning.

Before I go any further, I want to be sure to mention that learning takes *many* forms, and that there's more to it than reading. I am not of the camp that believes everyone needs to go to college. While I am troubled by the declining numbers of young men enrolling in and graduating from college, I also acknowledge that there are many reasons for that. Our culture would do well to encourage boys and young men to pay more attention to other potential paths, including military service, as well as trades like electrical maintenance, carpentry, plumbing, transportation, and construction. Richard Reeves, whose research I mentioned earlier, has offered some insightful recommendations about alternatives to college—specifically apprenticeships—that might provide ideal paths for young men to pursue.[6]

Regardless of whether young men are pursuing college or some other vocational path, though, we have to be careful not to fall into the same trap that much of our culture does, which is to draw some artificial distinction between "intellectual" men and "real" men. Our contemporary cultural narrative has succeeded to some extent in portraying the arts, for example, as inherently feminine pursuits—and that reductive mentality is not good for men or women. Spending time in the intellectual playground isn't mutually exclusive of "non-intellectual" endeavors, whether you're a college guy or not. You can be an electrician *and* study Aristotle. You can go hard at football *and* lose yourself in poetry. You can be into hunting *and* be fascinated by geometry. You can love both comic books *and* Shakespeare.

It's (apparently) controversial to suggest it, but I think one of the things that would help this situation for boys is to have more male teachers. The K–12 teaching workforce is overwhelmingly female, and that may suggest something to boys about who school is "for." Imagine how the educational landscape might be different for boys if they had a more balanced combination of men *and* women teaching them, and saw both as embodying what it means to teach and learn. At the private high school for boys where I teach, for example, the breakdown is roughly 50 percent male teachers and 50 percent female—and I think our young men benefit from that balance of faculty influence.

ACTIVE LEARNING

Just as strength, courage, and discipline are important parts of masculinity, so too are intellectual curiosity and deep thinking. What does it mean to think? And how often do we let ourselves really do it? This is sort of a meta-exercise, to ask you to think about thinking. But let's try.

Deep thinking is immersive. It means you get involved in ideas and let your imagination play around with them. If you make your thinking immersive, it'll let you find adventure in any kind of learning—whether it's learning how to snowboard, fix an engine, or comprehend the intricacies of literature.

I'm sure it's not hard to see how you could find adventure in learning to snowboard. But as an English teacher and a lover of stories, I know you can find great adventure in reading, too. I want to spend a little time on it, precisely for the reason I described earlier—that it seems boys and men are getting away from reading.

There is so much guys can get from reading. Reading can be inspiring. It can help us see that the world is bigger than our own problems. And that's a powerful force that can work against the anxiety and depression that are so present among young guys these days. If you don't think reading is for you, go to a bookstore and look around. Find something that fascinates you. There are a lot of books out there, on anything you can imagine.

The key is to get immersed. I teach the guys in my class to immerse themselves in what they're learning, like a swimmer diving into a pool. When they're reading a book or article, for example, I challenge them to use a simple, three-step process:

1. Notice.

2. Reflect.

3. Respond.

I said the process is *simple*, not *easy*. The first part is the hardest. You have to put yourself in a position to *notice stuff*. Sounds simple enough, but distractions are everywhere. You have to be intentional about putting your phone away, or at least on do not disturb. That's *really hard* for some of us to do. Noticing also requires you to slow down long enough to picture what you're reading and to detect things that you might not see if you're going fast or if you're trying to multitask by thinking about something else.

What do you notice? Anything, really. The unique words that a character uses. The way an author describes an approaching thunderstorm. Patterns of behavior that tip us off to what might happen in later chapters. This is like noticing a new structure on the playground, realizing how cool it is, and allowing yourself to get a little excited as you imagine what it would actually feel like to go climb on it. It's like surveying the terrain.

The second part, "reflect," is important. Questions are an essential part of thinking. In a lot of ways, questions are even more important than answers, because they spur you to the kind of mental action required to achieve those answers. It's in this mental action of searching that real thinking happens.

So, what is reflection? When you reflect on something, you think back on it in a questioning way. Noticing reveals the "who, what, where, when, and how" of what you read or experience. But reflection calls for two more elements: "why, and so what?" It's examining the significance of what has happened—the significance to you, to others, and to the course of life. By reflecting this way, you take a good look at what's happened, and really begin to understand things a little better.

Questioning can be critical, when it involves pushing, poking, prodding, and asking, "What if?" and "Yeah, okay, but what about this?" If noticing is looking hard and listening to what you're reading, then questioning is pushing back a little. It's looking more closely at that terrain. Turning over rocks. Looking for patterns.

Questioning helps you identify what isn't clear. You make a note in the margins of the book that says, "I don't get this. What does this mean?" There's value in expressing a question, even if the answer isn't apparent. Reflective questions make you think. They remind you there's more to learn.

Reflection is exploring; it is trying something out you haven't done before. What if I go on the big slide? What if I try climbing that thing? Can I make it all the way across the monkey bars? Is that really as scary as it looks? Man, that looks like fun! What would it feel like if I made it to the top of that thing? What if I fell from there?

The next part is "respond." Having an emotional response is a way of responding. Really letting yourself *feel* something. Maybe something you read makes you anxious, angry, or frustrated; maybe it makes you laugh or feel some sort of relief, or it brings you joy.

Another response is praise or criticism. Maybe a particular sentence is just really well written or an idea is especially compelling. On the other hand, maybe something the author has said seems purely idiotic, hypocritical, or just downright wrong. Maybe it gets you fired up. That's good! Get excited! Get fired up! Let yourself feel what you feel when you're learning something. Then express it! In the case of a book, *write* something. If you page through the books owned by people who have made a habit of actively reading, you'll see margins full of notes. They've made their books just as messy as life itself.

For some guys, the most adventurous part of responding to a book is talking about it, arguing about it, and debating about it. Responding is among the most exciting parts of being on the playground. It's pushing the boundaries. It's reveling in the thrill of climbing, falling, swinging, bouncing. It's deciding what you like to do and what was boring, it's experiencing the full range of playground feelings—excitement, fear, anticipation, exhilaration, boredom, joy, and the sharpening of your competitive edge.

Of course, reading books is only *one* arena of thinking and learning. You can apply the same process of noticing, questioning, and responding to virtually every aspect of your daily life.

This is a pretty useful way of thinking deeply about a problem, an idea, an event, a question, a challenge, a consequence, a person, a place, a relationship, an investment, a risk, etc. The list goes on. In each case, using the methodology of *notice, question, respond* will involve getting in deep.

And when you get in deep—when you let your mind and heart really engage with something intellectual—it becomes part of your pilgrimage. It becomes part of your adventure.

FREEING YOURSELF TO THINK

Deep thinking takes time.

You can't multitask and do this kind of immersive thinking and reflection. You have to disconnect and allow yourself time and space to think—that is, *just* to think. Take a second to think about how often you really just let yourself think! When was the last time you took time to do *nothing* but sit in a chair, or lie down in the grass, or go for a walk, and just *think*?

Of course, we usually have to do our thinking while we do other things, because that's life. We can't spend hours each day staring up at the sky and letting our thoughts run freely.

Also, it's no secret that sometimes doing something else *can* enhance our thinking. Having a meaningful conversation with your best friend can expand your mind, deepen your own sense of your soul at work, at play, discovering the world. Talking can be a playful form of thinking.

Even a respectful argument can get you going. If you've ever taken a class that used Socratic discussion methods (back-

and-forth dialogue, including debate), you know the excitement of quick thinking and good comebacks.

Two other ways of just sitting and thinking and, thus, *feeling your thoughts*, are through music and exercise. Listening to music or going for a walk can be very conducive to thinking. Literally, because like electricity, they "conduct" cells throughout your brain, and those cells take you to new places physically, if you are walking, and neurologically, if you are just listening to a song and mirroring it in your brain.

The point here is that you have to be intentional about thinking. You have to see the value of investing time, energy, and focus. Be as intentional about it as you are about eating or exercising. But watch out, because there are pitfalls in thinking, just like in anything else.

THE DANGER OF REDUCTIVE THINKING

One of the most dangerous pitfalls is what I'll call "reductive thinking." It means jumping to conclusions about cause and effect.

I coached a kid—let's call him Steve—who began struggling in school right about the same time he joined the crew team. Steve's grades were slipping quite a bit, and his parents expressed concern that it had to do with the three hours of practice every day. They pulled him from the team, assuming the increased time for study would bring his grades back up. You can guess what happened next, right?

His grades got worse, instead. On top of the academic problems, he also became sullen, bored, and angry. I talked to Steve's parents and explained the research that has shown most boys do better when engaged with athletics and extracurriculars, despite the time they consume.

He came back, and his grades improved. Eventually, we had a follow-up conference with his parents, teachers, and his counselor. Through his tears, Steve explained what had caused the original slip in his grades. It became clear it was totally unrelated to school or rowing—it was a falling out he'd had with a close friend. It just happened to occur around the same time he joined the team.

Steve's parents had assumed that the cause of his academic troubles lay with his busy schedule. It was a logical assumption, but it was incorrect. In fact, the attempted solution actually made things worse. It's dangerous to jump to conclusions.

Assuming we know the cause of something keeps us from considering other possibilities. This is reductive thinking. It's what happens when we look at a complicated situation and oversimplify what caused it—in the worst case, we hone in on one causal factor to the exclusion of all the others. You saw this kind of oversimplification happen in the example with Steve. Let's consider a different example.

Say there are four high school swim teams, which we'll call teams A, B, C, and D. Team B has its own on-campus pool and the other three don't. Team B—the one with its own pool—is consistently stronger, year after year, and has come in first place in the league for seven of the past ten years. A single cause interpretation would be, "Well, of course. It's because team B has a huge advantage. They have their own pool."

Except there could be any number of reasons why team B performs better. Maybe having their own pool is, in fact, the key to their success, and if you took it away their results would be weaker. On the other hand, it could have nothing to do with it at all. Maybe they simply train more effectively, year after year. Maybe they have stronger athletes, year after year. Maybe they have a better coach. In fact, maybe their on-campus pool is actually a *disadvantage*, because the heating system is lousy and it's always a little too cold.

There are two big problems with oversimplifying the cause of something. The first is that it's just lazy; it doesn't require much thought. The second is that it can lead to bad decisions. What if the league decided the other three teams should have some sort of handicap? Or that team B should have limits imposed on how much practice time it gets?

Either of these policy decisions might be very attractive to some people, because they might *seem* fair at first glance. The problem is that they are both based on reductive interpretations of what are actually complex sets of causes.

The Trap of Binary Thinking

A potentially serious obstacle to free thought is an extreme form of reductive thought: binary thinking. It's a trap we often fall into.

Binary thinking assumes everything is either one thing or its opposite. Everything is black or white—no shades of gray. Binary thinking makes people ignore the fact that two truths can (and often do) exist simultaneously. To be clear, I'm not saying that binaries don't exist. I don't think *everything* exists on a spectrum. The lights are either on or off. There's a winner and a loser in a football game. But many things depend on the circumstances. For example, you might support something under one set of circumstances, but not under another. Or you might agree with some of an argument, but not all of it.

Very often, binary thinking comes from getting in too deep with an ideology—a set of beliefs and corresponding attitudes. Ideologies aren't necessarily bad. But a reductive ideology is dangerous. It prescribes a narrow-minded set of scripted answers to very complex questions.

This is often what happens when people become true idealogues. In ways large and small, they stop thinking for themselves and instead gradually become mouthpieces for ideological talking points—which, of course, thrive on simplistic thinking. This is perhaps most obvious when it comes to politics. If you've ever had a truly frustrating discussion with someone who leans very far in one direction on a political spectrum, you know it's hard to even get that person to *think* about an opposing perspective, let alone consider its merits.

Our experiences online can reinforce reductive thinking by tailoring our online environment so that we hear more of what we want to hear. It's a self-perpetuating problem. Echo chambers get louder because of how social media algorithms work.

Hardcore reductive ideologues are easy to spot. They talk a lot, they repeat the same things other idealogues say, and they don't really listen. They aren't interested in thinking about what anyone else has to say. They really can't stand it when you answer their questions with, "Well, it depends." They don't like the complexity that response acknowledges. They want your answer neater and cleaner. They want it to fit in their ideological box.

Please don't misunderstand me. I'm not suggesting you should never stand on principle. I'm not suggesting that you shouldn't take positions on important matters or that everything is simply relativistic. What I am saying is that it's vitally important to acknowledge complexities and incorporate them in your positions. You can stand firmly on a principle while also acknowledging that the opposing viewpoint may have merit, too. Reasonable people can disagree on things. It's part of what enables society to function. Hell, it's what enables friendship to function, not to mention marriage. Any relationship, really.

Be very careful if you find yourself surrounded by ideologues. If you are, it's probably time to get out of the echo chamber. Echo chambers can take a lot of forms—a group chat, a social media channel, a news source, a political party, a celebrity fan club, an athletic team, a locker room, or a lunch table. Sometimes even families can become ideological echo chambers.

If you find *yourself* falling into the trap of a reductive ideology, political or otherwise, be careful. It'll discourage you from thinking outside of a narrow set of ideas about the world. That is not helpful on the path. Of course, the true value of taking a "both/and" approach to thinking is that it helps you achieve balance in everyday life. Consider these different ways of looking at matters of everyday life:

"I can either work hard enough *or* get enough sleep. I can't do both."

"I can work hard *and* get sufficient sleep."

—

"You're either with me *or* against me."

"I can disagree with your opinion *and* respect both it and you."

—

"I can either be healthy *or* I can eat unhealthy snacks; not both."

"I can maintain a healthy diet *and* enjoy occasional unhealthy snacks."

—

"I can put my efforts into school or sports; not both."

"I can work hard at both my academics *and* my athletics."

"I can't support x because there's one thing x does/says that I disagree with."

"I can be a part of x *and* disagree with some of its positions."

For each set of statements, ask yourself: Which seems more sustainable and practical? Which speaker would you want as a friend or teammate? How about as a college roommate? Which would you want as a business partner? Which one would you want to hire if you were a boss? Here's a kicker: which person would you want to marry?

Knowledge, Experience, and Understanding

True learning involves knowledge, experience, and understanding. These are three different things. Knowledge is stuff that you know. Experience is stuff that you've done. Understanding is having a grasp of the significance of knowledge and experience, and then being able to use it in some meaningful way.

Consider learning how to tie some knots. That's one thing I still remember from the Coast Guard Academy. First, you need some fundamental knowledge: the necessary information. This includes terms like knot, rope, tension, taut, loop, slack, slip, etc.

Next, you need some experience. You need to practice, and that involves messing up and succeeding. As you combine the knowledge with experience, you build your understanding:

what types of knots are best for different purposes, materials, and circumstances.

The cool thing is, you can continue to deepen your understanding of anything indefinitely. Even if you spend a lifetime learning everything there is to know about knots—I mean *everything* there is to know—and you have years and years of experience tying them, you continually combine your knowledge and experience of knots with your knowledge and experience of other things to understand other things in different ways.

The problem is, if you never make the decision to set out to learn about tying knots in the first place, well, the rest of the process I just described never gets a chance to follow, does it? So, yeah, we have to be intentional about learning.

INNOVATIVE LEADERS NEVER LEAVE THE PLAYGROUND

If you want to be a leader, be a lifelong learner.

People who are open to growth, who avoid reductive thinking, and who avoid falling into the trap of binary thinking have the qualities needed to be inspiring, innovative leaders.

Aiming for excellence as we make our path demands that we be true thinkers and learners. If we want to make the best path we can, then we need to stretch the limits of what we know, experience, and understand. We have to be humble enough to acknowledge that there's always more to learn. We have to be willing to be changed by learning—that's part of being open to growth.

Share the fact that you're reading this book. And then go read other books. Find other people to talk about them with. Don't shy away from books and reading because society implies these pursuits aren't manly. (And hey, pro tip, just in case you happen to be trying to meet women: Join a book club. You'll probably be one of the only guys there.)

Surely, you know the ancient Socratic maxim that "the unexamined life is not worth living." Those are strong words, sure, but I think Socrates was extending a strong admonishment to anyone who would dare to take the phenomenal learning opportunity that is life for granted.

He suggested that the moment we stop being open to growth, we stop living purposefully.

He encouraged us to dwell always in the playground of the intellect. Always to explore, to try, to test, to reflect, to push, to know, to understand, and to learn. To be courageous in the face of danger, because we might fall down and get hurt. But more than anything, to embrace the adventure that is lifelong learning.

Never leave the playground.

CHAPTER SEVEN

Telos

Developing a Life Vision

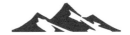

"JIMMY" WAS A HEFTY KID. When he showed up on day one of preseason training on a humid August morning, he stood out from the rest of the freshmen. At fourteen, he was very overweight. I was well into my coaching career by the time I met him, and I'd seen some out-of-shape kids before. But Jimmy was at a different level. I wondered if he'd stick with it. He was understandably self-conscious among the other boys, most of whom seemed more naturally athletic. By comparison, they were lean, strong, and agile.

We started with a one-mile "cycle run." I knew this was good practice for the opening session, because it kept the group together. In a cycle run, everyone jogs in a single-file column. You put a pacesetter at the front. The last guy in the back steps out to the side and sprints to the front of the column, slowing to match the pacesetter. The cycle continues for the duration of the run. Effectively, it's an interval workout. You can adjust the difficulty by spacing out the column or the speed of the jogging pace.

That time, I ran up front, slightly off to the side, and set the pace. I kept it pretty slow for day one. I wanted everyone to finish. In fact, we were going slow enough that I could mostly jog backwards and keep an eye on the group. A few guys who seemed in pretty good shape joked about the easy pace. The joking stopped after a few cycles of interval sprints.

It took most of the boys about eight or ten seconds to sprint to the front. Jimmy took almost half a minute, and it was not what you would call a sprint. He could barely accelerate. He had to plod forward, pushing hard, breathing hard, and slowly inching past each guy in the column. I was on the lookout for laughter or wisecracks, but nobody made so much as a quip. I think they were awestruck at his effort.

At the end of practice, we ended with a cool-down stretch. Afterward, Jimmy came up to me and asked if I thought he could do this. I answered his question with another question: I asked him why he *wanted* to do this. He said he wanted to be an athlete. He was tired of being overweight and out of shape. The way he said it—the look of determination in his eyes—made it clear: Jimmy had a vision. But he needed a plan.

The Difference between a Vision and a Plan

I've said this to students for years: "Figure out a long-term vision. It'll see you through the errors of your attempted long-term planning." Making a good path requires both vision and plans—but the order matters. If you form a vision first—a sense of what you're aiming for, and a good understanding of why—then it will guide your plans for how to get there. On the other hand, if you start making plans without a clear vision, you stand a good chance of getting lost or confused. Here are some examples of visions:

"I want to be a man of integrity."

"I want to be a generous leader."

"I want to be a loving husband and father."

Notice that these aren't complicated statements. They aren't mired in specific details. That's on purpose! Having a vision for your life just means knowing and understanding what *kind* of man you want to be, and what *kind* of life you want to live— and knowing *why*. Living out a vision does require planning, but it also depends on being adaptable and understanding that plans have to change.

The title of this chapter is another Greek word: *telos*, which means, basically, "end goal." If you consider the word "telescope," you can see the connection. A telescope is an instrument that allows us to see things from very far away. That's exactly how long-term vision should seem when you're a young guy: a long way off.

SHORT-TERM VISIONS AND PLANS

Visions and plans are useful in the shorter term, too. Let's say you want to build better strength. That's a vision. Once you have it, you can develop a training plan. Maybe you talk to a trainer, or you do some research online to figure out how to realize your vision. You develop a specific training schedule, and you stick to it. That's a plan.

Take a guy who wants to get better at math. He has a vision of himself with a better understanding of math principles. He imagines a version of himself who doesn't break out in a cold sweat at the beginning of math class every day. Then he develops a plan: "Visit with my teacher twice per week, commit to a half hour of study and practice per night, and see a tutor until my average reaches eighty-five."

Maybe you're shy and not very confident talking to people. You freeze up. You have a vision of a more confident version of yourself—not a different guy, but just more confident. So you make a plan. You pick three people you trust of whom you can ask advice. You commit to reading a few articles, from intelligent websites, about how to build confidence. Then you commit to taking the plunge—you're going to try to strike up one new conversation each day, in a time or place where you normally wouldn't have tried.

If you've been paying attention, you may have noticed a couple distinctions between visions and plans. The first is that visions are pretty general. Visions are about who we want to be and what we want to do generally. Plans are the *specifics* of how we intend to get there. The second distinction is that visions are about what we *desire*, and plans are about how we're going to *achieve* what we desire. This means it's really important to figure out what we *truly* desire. More on that soon.

Vision and planning depend on each other. Visions without plans don't go anywhere. Plans without vision are probably going to fall apart, because they aren't carefully aimed.

LONG-TERM VISION (TELOS) AND PLANS

The examples we just considered might play out over a period of weeks or months. Now let's shift to long term, the telos. If you want to aim for excellence and make a good path, it's important to have a long-term vision for your life. Maybe you think you're too young to form a vision.

Nope.

You might be too young to make a long-term *plan* for your life. But if you're old enough to be reading a book like this, you're old enough to begin developing a long-term *vision*. You can (and should) begin forming a vision for your life as a teenager.

In fact, I think if a guy hasn't at least begun to define a vision for his life by the time he's in his late teens, he's probably in for some trouble. Remember—there's a difference between *forming* a vision and *achieving* it.

Vision, as I mentioned, is what sustains us when our plans have to change or when they fall apart. (And they do.) On the other hand, planning can help when vision fails, but it probably won't be enough. It can keep things from going completely to hell, at least temporarily, but without a solid vision, all the plans in the world won't amount to much for very long.

Both visions and plans can be exciting, and they can both be intimidating. If you think about it, though, a vision tends to be a little less intimidating than a plan. The vision is aspirational, while the plan is definitive. The vision is like a soft voice, encouraging, saying, "Take your time to get here. You can do it."

My grandfather was a visionary, to me. His soft but firm voice captured, without complaint, the trials and tribulations of all his life planning toward realizing his visions. His eye focused on telos for a long, long time, and then, in his old age, he could look back and see how visionary he had been, and how well (and sometimes not well) his plans had worked.

If grandpa was the visionary, the plan is, to me, the drill sergeant. The plan is the prodding voice that says, "Do *this*, *now*. Get ready to do *this*, next!" We all need the drill sergeant, the motivator, the one who keeps us in line and following the plan. But we should never forget the visionary, the softer voice in the background as we follow the plan, the one saying, "Here's why you are doing all this, because you are on a pilgrim's journey, growing your soul."

How Vision Helps You Deal with Fear

We need both voices, but there's a problem if we get so used to that drill sergeant voice that we can't hear the softer but equally important grandpa. When this happens to you, sit back and wonder whether you have fallen into a trap we all fall into, where your primary motivator is now your own fear of failure.

Fear is always with us as men. It's not wrong or bad to be afraid. Courage is not the absence of fear, after all—it's the willingness to confront it. Fear can be a useful motivator. For me, for instance, when I feel afraid that I'm not making enough of a living to provide for my family, I work even harder at my job. When I fear that I made a mistake with my wife or kids, I am motivated to apologize or otherwise fix the problem. Fear of error, or falling behind, or not fulfilling expectations . . . these fears are fine.

But if fear is the only thing motivating you, you're going to get exhausted. In that case, things will likely not go so well for you, especially when you are grappling internally with a fear of failure, a deep sense of inadequacy, that you must recognize. Around me I see young guys scared, a lot of the time, who don't realize how unnecessarily scared they are.

They're scared of seeming inadequate. They're scared of being left behind and excluded from the groups they admire and respect. They're scared of disappointing their families. They're afraid that by failing to earn some specific achievement—maybe something they don't even really care about—they'll be regarded as failures overall.

Have you seen them, too?

Are you one of them?

They're scared and anxious about uncertainties and about failing in part because they're more focused on their plans than their vision.

In my own life, when I face a problem, I try to envision what things could look like if I handle it right. When I do that, the fear goes away, or at least diminishes enough that I will not be paralyzed by it. Let's say I have a nasty argument with my wife. It leaves me feeling fearful and stuck. What do I do? I see myself—I envision myself, that is—talking to her about it and apologizing. After the vision has helped me quiet my fear, I am able to plan out next steps, when to approach her, what to say that allows me to keep my dignity (because, hey, I was not *totally* wrong, after all!), and heal the rift with her.

The vision shows me what I'm aiming for. It also shows me I'm capable of doing it, and that helps greatly to quiet my fear of failure. Then I can plan what to do.

Clarify your vision before making your plan. A lot of guys expend huge amounts of energy trying to make long-term plans *before* they've clarified their vision. The loss of energy comes from the plan failing a lot. It's hard to make a plan for a *day* that doesn't end up having to change. Why should we assume we can reliably plan for a period of years, let alone a lifetime, without having a clear vision? Vision quiets our fear of failure and frees us to make a good path.

The College Fear, and the Career Telos

When I talk with juniors and seniors in high school, I hear a lot of anxiety about the next steps on their path. Since I teach at a college prep school, most of the guys are planning on college. Every year there are a handful who don't and instead enlist in the military, pursue a trade school, or take a gap year. But most are headed to college. So, the questions surround where to go, what to study, what job options will emerge, and what salary range is likely.

For many of them, at the core of all this anxiety lies a simple fear: *what if I can't make it?* So I ask them, "*Why* do you want to go to college?" The response is nearly always formulaic: to earn a degree that makes me a viable job candidate who will make a viable salary so I can be self-sufficient . . . and so it goes on. That's all well and good, because it's true. That formulaic approach to answering the question certainly isn't wrong.

But it does beg another question: Have you thought about what *kind* of life you want to live, and what *kind* of man you want to be as you live your life? That's the big question, I think. That's the important *desire* to figure out: what kind of man do you want to be?

Maybe college isn't even the right next step at all.

Of course, if you're a little older, you might be looking at the same fears and questions from a different perspective. Maybe you're past the "college fears," but now you've got the same questions about the early steps in your career.

The good news is that no matter how old we are, the same wisdom applies. Vision and planning are interdependent. You've got to start with telos. You've got to start with the long-term vision before you can build an effective plan.

Turns out there's an app for that.

An ancient, time-tested one.

A Formula for Making Visions and Plans

"Begin with the end in mind." This is an ancient educational idea, but it was rephrased for a whole generation of business leaders by author Stephen Covey in *The 7 Habits of Highly Effective People*, which has sold many millions of copies since its publication in 1989.[1] I didn't go to business school, but teachers have to begin with the end in mind, too. If I begin designing an English course by just listing a bunch of books I want my students to read, I'm in trouble.

A couple of veteran educators, Grant Wiggins and Jay McTighe, came up with a great model for designing courses called "backward design."[2] If you're rolling your eyes, I don't blame you. But bear with me. I promise this is useful—because you can adapt this model to develop a vision and a plan for your life. "Backward design" comes down to three simple steps:

1. Define the goal. What should students know, and why? What should they understand about that knowledge, and why?

2. Figure out how you'll measure success. How will I know if students have gained this knowledge and understanding?

3. Make a plan. What course content will I use? How and when?

Okay. What does this look like if you apply it to your life, instead of a course?

1. Where are you going? Where do you want your path to take you—and why? (That's your vision! Your telos! Your aim!)

2. How will you know you're getting closer, and when you've arrived? (Those are your milestones!)

3. How will you get there? What specific action steps will you take, and in what sequence? (That's your plan!)

We can apply these three questions to both short-term and long-term contexts. Let's go back to the example of building strength.

1. I want my path to take me to greater strength, because I want to be more capable and confident with my body.

2. I'll know if I've arrived based on some specific strength tests and whether I feel more confident.

3. I'm going to do x workouts, x days per week, for x weeks, making slight adjustments based on my progress.

You can see where it would be tempting to just have a general goal of getting ripped, look up some workouts online, and go hit the gym. While that might work, you can see the benefit of defining the telos first—of figuring out precisely what it is you want and *why* you want it. You might say, "But it's so obvious why." Don't be so sure. It's one thing just to say, "I want to get stronger." It's another thing entirely to say,

"I want to get stronger because I want to be more capable and confident with my body."

Because here's the thing: If you only state your vision the first way, without clarifying *why*, then you're more likely to give up on it when the going gets tough. If you take some time to figure out exactly *why* you want to do something, you'll probably be better at sticking with it. This will also help you notice if you're being motivated by fear. For example, is your motivation actually to be stronger and more confident, or is it really more that you are driven by the fear and insecurity of being smaller than other guys? That's important to know, because there will always be someone bigger and stronger—so that fear isn't necessarily going to be helpful.

You've heard the term "beach muscles," right? Beach muscles make a guy look strong—and, to be fair, they probably mean he *is* strong, at least in some ways. However, having big, strong biceps, for example, doesn't add a great deal of functional capability—especially if a guy doesn't develop adequate core strength to go with them. Then again, if your telos is looking bro-tastic in tank tops at concerts, then you'd be right on, man. But be careful. Don't skip leg day.

If you look back up at those three questions, you'll see that they are each interconnected with the other two. So, what does all that mean? It means that when it comes to vision and planning, all three components are important—because each depends upon the other.

Vision and Planning Depend on Each Other

If we want our plans to get us anywhere, they need to be oriented at a telos. It's good if that telos involves aiming for excellence.

We know that means clarifying a vision. But that can be hard to figure out. So how do we figure out what we *truly* desire? That's where something called "discernment" comes in, and that's the focus of the next chapter.

—◆—

Remember Jimmy? Well, the kid had a vision but lacked a plan. He knew that, and he came to our team looking for a plan. He listened to his coaches, and he stuck to the regimen, day after day, month after month. When something wasn't working, he modified his approach.

He lost a lot of excess weight over the course of his first year rowing. Over the next three, he continued to slim down, even as his body grew and developed. Eventually, he won championship races. By the time he graduated, he looked like a different person. The change was more than physical, though. It showed in the way he carried himself. He was more confident. He was happy.

CHAPTER EIGHT

Discernment and Authentic Desires

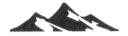

I HAVE A GUMMY BEAR PROBLEM. Well, not just gummy bears, really, but all gummy candy. Left unsupervised in the presence of the colorful little treasures, it is entirely likely that I will consume several hundred calories in ten minutes.

They call those one-pound bags "share size."

Not a chance, bucko. Those are all mine.

I keep them hidden from my children. Guilty as charged.

I like the clear ones best.

Yes, I have a gummy bear problem.

But see, I also like being in good shape. Back in high school, I was the captain of the rowing and swimming teams, and I had a body fat percentage somewhere in the low single digits. I had a six-pack. I swear I did. Even now, I work out pretty regularly, and I'm in "okay" shape for a middle-aged guy. I don't have a six-pack anymore, though. Which is okay, because I don't care so much about the six-pack at this point in my life. But to be sure, my desire to be in good shape is a deeper, more firmly rooted, more *authentic* desire than my desire to consume excessive quantities of gummy candy.

LIMITS CAN SET US FREE

Remember our discussion of virtue? We said that we need rules, at least at first, to create good habits. Well, rules have another benefit. They help us figure out what we truly want.

In order to say "yes" to our most authentic desires, we have to be able to say "no" to other, competing desires. We are most free to pursue our most authentic desires when we restrict ourselves in some way.

That's right: limits can actually *create* freedom. Kind of a paradox, right? But it's true. By saying no to gummy bears, I'm effectively saying yes to better health and better physical shape.

Think of a traffic light. It helps us get places. How? It enables us to *go* by making us *stop*. Or, more precisely, it enables some cars to go by making others stop on an alternating basis. You could say, then, that the red light is just as much a part of "going" as the green light is. You can't get a green light without red lights involved.

Paradoxically enough, then, red lights are the key to reaching our destination in one piece. If I want to achieve my deeper desire of being healthy and looking decent without my shirt on (six-pack or not) then clearly, I need some red lights when it comes to gummy bears. Limits help us control our cravings, so we can stay on a path that follows our *genuine* desires.

Okay, so that makes sense in terms of fighting off temptations and cravings: The gummy bear path is tempting, but the healthy path is obviously better. But what about a situation where we have to *choose between two good paths?* Discernment can help us there, and we can look to the wisdom of a saint to learn how to go about it.

Saint Ignatius Loyola

Ignatius of Loyola, a Catholic saint, was born in 1491 in the Basque region of Spain. A dashing, charismatic nobleman, he was ambitious, bold, and quite the ladies' man. Then he underwent a powerful spiritual conversion after having his leg decimated by a cannonball in battle. Stuck in a room recovering for a long time, he got pretty bored. The Wi-Fi was terrible. His best bet was reading. He wanted stories of glorious adventure and worldly conquest. To his dismay, he had access only to the Bible and some stories about the saints. With nothing else to do, he cracked them open and got reading.

He began to notice something over the course of the days and weeks. Whenever he imagined a future of bold, daring adventure full of romance and fame—the kinds of things he'd fantasized about throughout his youth—he found himself feeling kind of empty. But then, when he imagined a life trying to emulate the saints he was reading about—a life without worldly glory—he felt a sort of peaceful, encouraging joy. He figured out that by really zooming in on his feelings, by becoming carefully attuned to how different visions made him *feel*, he could understand himself on a deeper level. He was able to form a vision truly in keeping with his deepest, most genuine desires. This discovery of his ability to *discern* authentic desires from less substantial cravings or passing desires was, in a sense, the beginning of his spiritual journey.

Ignatius eventually went on to found the Society of Jesus, better known as the Jesuits. This is the religious order to which Pope Francis belongs, and it has become the largest order in the Church, with about sixteen thousand priests and brothers. I've spent my career teaching in Jesuit high schools, and education is one of the Jesuits' most important missions. I'm telling you about Saint Ignatius not because this is a book about spirituality or religion, but because his teachings and writings, as articulated in his *Spiritual Exercises*, have inspired one of the most influential spiritual traditions in the world. The *Spiritual Exercises* provides an experience of meditative prayer, personal reflection, and directed conversation—all rooted largely in something called the "discernment of spirits."

Discernment, Consolation, and Desolation

For Ignatius, discernment involved becoming carefully attuned, through meditative prayer, honest conversation, and deep reflection, to the way various things made him feel. This became especially relevant when he had an important decision to make— what to do, whom to follow, which of two possibilities to pursue.

He found this was especially useful when either option could be a good one. Generally, he found, one option or possibility would give him a sense of wholeness, of being on the right track, of purposeful "rightness" and of peace—even if there were unanswered questions. He called the combination of these feelings "consolation." On the other hand, some options or possibilities would give rise to a combination of feelings he called "desolation": emptiness, unease, anxiety, hopelessness, discouragement—a general sense of "wrong-ness." I think it's helpful to look at consolation and desolation side by side like this, with a list of the contrasting feelings each involves:

Consolation		Desolation
Peaceful		Anxious or conflicted
Hopeful		Hopeless
Clarity		Confusion
True, genuine		False, deceptive
Free to change and grow	← vs →	Trapped, confined, or paralyzed
Full		Empty
Balanced		Excess or lack
Healthy solitude		Lonely isolation
Reconciliation		Shame or resentment
Grateful		Unappreciative

THE EXAMEN: A WAY OF DISCERNMENT

So, what is discernment like? How can you put it into daily practice as you make your path? Well, whether you want to think of it as prayer or simply as meditation, it boils down to developing a habit of reflection about your own daily experiences. We discussed reflection a couple chapters back, remember? It's examining the significance of what has happened—the significance to me, to others, and to the course of life.

For Ignatius, this took the form of a meditative prayer practice he called the "Examination of Conscience," variably referred to as the "Examination of Consciousness," but which is now more commonly known simply as the "the Examen." It can be done at any time throughout the day, but I think it makes sense to try to stick to a regular time, like in the quiet of the morning or the evening before going to bed. This is best achieved in a quiet space, without distractions, but it can also be done while you're walking the dog, raking leaves, or out for a run or bike ride. It goes like this:

1. Express gratitude to God for the day you've had and the opportunity to reflect upon it.

2. Ask for the honesty to see where you've messed up, or sinned. When did you do the wrong thing? Where did you fail to do the right thing? When were you not the guy you really want to be?

3. Review the day you've had, recalling what happened and how it made you feel. Consider how different moments provided you with feelings of consolation and desolation.

4. Express remorse for the times when you messed up today. Ask God for forgiveness for your sins.

5. Express gratitude again for the experiences of the day, and resolve to strive to do better tomorrow.

Obviously, Saint Ignatius was religious. He has had such a big impact on the Christian spiritual tradition that his teachings and practices have come to be called "Ignatian Spirituality." He believed our most authentic desires line up with God's desires for us. If we live our life truly attuned to our *most authentic* desires—not the false ones, as deceptive as they may be—we will live in accord with God and realize the full goodness of God's hopes and desires for us. Sounds pretty good, right?

Of course, even if you aren't religious, you can still find value in the process of discernment. You can still benefit greatly from careful attention to feelings of consolation and desolation when you're trying to make a difficult decision. Because of my faith, when I do the Examen, I consider it a prayerful conversation with God. If you prefer to take God out of the equation, you can still engage in reflective meditation using this approach. Just think of it as an honest conversation with *yourself*. And direct your gratitude wherever you wish—toward people or the world in general.

THE PRACTICALITY OF DISCERNMENT ON THE PATH

Consider the value of discernment as you try to make a good path. If you can engage in truly thoughtful, honest thinking about your conflicting desires, and be open to the way they make you feel at the deepest level, you'll be more attuned to yourself in a very useful way. If you aren't sure discernment applies to you, here are some examples of questions it could help you handle:

Is there something you do regularly in response to a temporary, shallow desire—but you know it runs contrary to a deeper, more meaningful desire? How does giving into it leave you feeling?

How do you decide between two good choices, such as whether to pursue one good opportunity or another? What do you think about? What feelings are involved—and do they play a role in your decision?

Is there a particular time, place, activity, or person (or some combination of those things) that consistently makes you feel especially "right" or "wrong"?

Those three questions are just sort of a starting exercise in the kind of reflective thinking at the core of discernment. In order to answer them honestly, you have to really *listen* to yourself and not go into the exercise favoring one answer over another. You can't trick yourself in the process of true discernment. And "no tricks" seems like a good policy for a guy trying to make a good path, right?

When you develop the ability to engage in true discernment, you become much more aware of your genuine desires. That doesn't mean you won't ever act on impulses and cravings—but you will probably be more aware of it. Hopefully, over time, you'll develop a better ability to resist those things *before* you do them. As you mature, when you're about to do or say something that runs contrary to those deeper desires, you'll get a little warning bell that says, "Hey man . . . that's not really what you want."

Maturity can be practiced. With practice, you will get better at listening to the warning bell and maintaining your discipline.

With practice, you'll get better at saying no to the gummy bears. With practice, you'll get better at seeing your own tendencies and habits, which will help you control them.

DISCERNING YOUR WAY TO DEEPER JOY

Of course, discernment isn't just about *not* taking bad steps that'll get us in trouble. More importantly, it's about taking good ones that lead us closer to being the guys we *genuinely* want to be in the depths of our hearts. You get better at saying "yes" to the true desires. When we do that, we walk a better path. We feel a sense of direction; we know our lives have meaning—and with that confidence comes great joy.

So, discernment can help us walk a joyful path, for sure. One of the reasons for that is that by helping us clarify our deepest, most authentic desires, it provides us with a point of reference for all the different aspects of our lives.

My challenge for you? Try doing the Examen every day.

I try to do it every morning. If I'm being honest, I don't always do it. But you know what? On the days that I do, I'm more focused and disciplined. I'm kinder to my family, colleagues, and students. I'm more at ease, yet I have more energy. I'm more patient, and I don't sweat the small stuff. I find greater joy in the ordinary stuff.

I'm closer to being the man I really want to be.

Oh . . . and I eat fewer gummy bears.

Try it. It works.

Chapter Nine

The Integrated Man

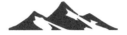

The *Vitruvian Man* is naked! When I projected the centuries-old image at the front of my ninth-grade English class, there was a tremor of laughter among the boys sitting at their desks in the darkened classroom. Of course, when I asked them to take an even closer look at it, it got even more awkward.

Because, well, the *Vitruvian Man* is naked.

I'm sure you've seen the image. It's the drawing of the guy standing with his arms and legs extended in two positions: first an X-shape, overlaid with a T-shape.

Once their fourteen-year-old brains adjusted to the image of a naked dude splayed across the eighty-five-inch projection screen and the nervous giggles worked themselves out, we were able to get into a good discussion.

After a while, we realized how the visual imagery of the drawing could help us understand the importance of balance and proportion when it comes to moral integrity. We were also able to consider what happens when we lack balance. It sure is hard to make a good path when things are out of balance.

THE BALANCED MAN

Vitruvius was a renowned Roman architect whose design principles inspired Leonardo da Vinci as he studied human anatomy. The now-famous image is a visual portrayal of what da Vinci had come to understand about the geometric proportions of the body.

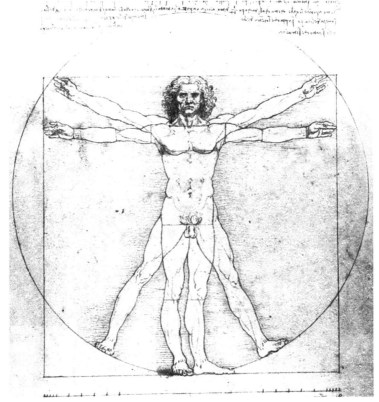

Detail of *Vitruvian Man* (c.1492) by Leonardo da Vinci. Drawing pen, ink and wash on paper. 34.6 × 25.5 cm. Gallerie dell'Accademia, Venice, Italy.
WIKIMEDIA COMMONS.

This might seem like strange territory for English class, but we were about to begin reading *Frankenstein* by Mary Shelley, and I wanted them to ponder a deep question: "What makes a man?" The themes of that novel relate to this existential matter; likewise, the story offers a wonderful exploration of the nature of obsession. I wanted my students to consider how passion (a healthy thing) can slide into obsession (not a healthy thing at all).

I wanted them to think about how excess can lead to imbalance. About how a man must maintain proportionality and balance in his life, or else both he and those around him might suffer. I wanted them to reflect upon how, as in *Frankenstein*, a lack of balance and proportionality might make a man into a monster—even as he produces other monsters, too.

As we dug deeper into the image of the *Vitruvian Man* in class, and putting predictable wisecracks about "ideal proportions" aside, the guys made some interesting observations. Among the most insightful was that the figure, while literally a model of balance, is neither perfectly symmetrical nor flawless. Perfection is not a prerequisite for balance or proportionality, and these ideals could be achieved despite our inevitable human flaws. Leonardo da Vinci could have applied the Renaissance equivalent of post-process photo editing to his image. Instead, he remained true to form.

After discussing balance and proportionality, we turned to their opposites: imbalance and disproportionality. Sometimes it's easiest to understand something by considering its opposite; in fact, sometimes we can *only* recognize something in relation to its opposite. Darkness is relative to light, for example. The lowered window shades in that classroom made it relatively dark, but compared to a *truly* dark basement with absolutely no light, it would hardly seem dark. Likewise, when I'm standing next to my wife, who is just barely five-two, I seem pretty tall, despite being only five-six.

As we talked about imbalance and disproportionality, we realized imbalance is both the cause *and* the effect of many human problems.

THE MONSTER MAN

Shelley's novel tells the story of a brilliant Swiss medical doctor, Victor Frankenstein, who becomes captivated by the power of electricity and obsessed with using it to conquer death itself. After a series of increasingly gruesome experiments, Victor succeeds in reanimating a corpse. Horrified at his own success, Victor abandons the helpless, terrified creature.

Repulsed by his own grotesque appearance and shunned by everyone, the creature lives a tortured life of loneliness. He is intelligent, though, and eventually learns to speak and read. He learns of his maker and takes vengeance in a series of cruel, violent reprisals against Victor's family and friends.

Victor's passion for science, played out across years of rigorous, disciplined study and the courageous advancement of experimental medical procedures, is admirable. But when it tips the scales into obsession and becomes wildly imbalanced, things go bad.

Such imbalance is caused by too much of one thing, usually in combination with too little of something else. In Victor's case, an excess of self-confidence, ego, and ambition was coupled with a lack of humility—resulting in the tragic flaw the Greeks called *hubris*. His ambition reached toxic levels, and the result was catastrophic—both for him and for many others.

How did things go so wrong for Victor Frankenstein? His superior knowledge, combined with reckless ambition, went unchecked, despite the damage to his relationships. Victor became so intent on proving he *could* do something that he didn't adequately consider whether he *should*. It seems he let his mind take over everything and forgot to use his heart and soul in his decisions.

You could say that this imbalance came from a lack of structural integrity—or, to be more precise, moral integrity.

STRUCTURAL INTEGRITY; MORAL INTEGRITY

The *Vitruvian Man* is a portrait of balance and proportionality, his extremities situated within the geometric confines of the circle and the square. No excess or insufficiency. The result is a sort of architectural integrity. The human body is a remarkable anatomical achievement built for endurance, strength, and agility. It's a fitting vessel for the most sophisticated brain on the planet, a neurochemical miracle with processing power exponentially higher than that of even our most advanced supercomputers.

This ideal of proportionality looks pretty good on paper. Maintaining such balance in all aspects of our lives, given the various imperfections and general asymmetry of our character flaws, is not easy. We are prone to excesses of all kinds, whether they relate to our temperament, our biases, our habits, or our proclivity to consume massive quantities of gummy bears.

So how do we maintain balance?

The answer lies with integrity.

A building with structural integrity uses design principles to distribute and absorb forces while holding its form. That requires both strength and flexibility. Consider the world's tallest skyscrapers. They have incredibly deep foundations and comprise thousands of tons of steel and concrete built to sway in the wind and not fall over.

When it comes to a person, we can talk about moral integrity. Moral integrity means continuity of moral character under different circumstances. In other words, a man with integrity acts more or less the same, in terms of his values, regardless of whom he's with or what's going on. To get back to the skyscraper analogy: he maintains his firm foundation regardless of which way the winds are blowing. Sure, he might bend or sway just slightly so as to adapt to the circumstances, but at the core, his foundation holds firm.

Importantly, he also acts more or less the same in terms of moral behavior, whether or not others are watching. So, a good basic measure of our integrity is the degree to which we maintain our moral behavior when no one could or would know the difference.

That's very hard to do.

But looking at a sort of "blueprint" for integrity can help.

Just like a skillful architect interconnects the various parts of a building to provide structural integrity, you can *integrate* the various parts of your being. Let's say you have four aspects: *body*, your physical being; *mind*, your knowledge and understanding; *heart*, your emotions and relationships; and *soul*, your spiritual being.

The more these aspects overlap, the more integrated you are. The less they overlap, the less integrated. The more each aspect is in touch with the others, the easier it is to maintain balance in your life.

Take a look at the Venn diagram. You'll see the four aspects overlapping. You can look at any two and see an overlap. But the key is that *all four* overlap.

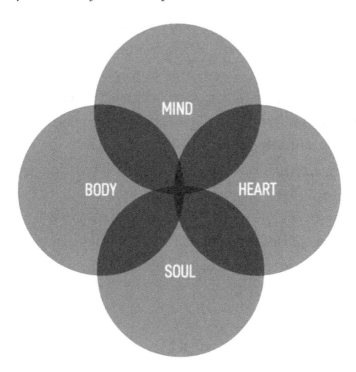

Mortal and Divine

One of the interesting takes on the *Vitruvian Man* involves the way it depicts this overlap by depicting our dual nature: mortal bodies with divine souls. If you look closely, the figure is centered within both a square and a circle. Within the circle, the man's limbs are extended like an "X," and the center point of the circle is the navel. This is the wellspring of life, where we begin, where we are connected to our mothers. Circles are a mystery. Like the divine, they have no beginning or end. They are, so to speak, the alpha and omega. They are infinite. Even the "number" we use to calculate the area of a circle, pi, is itself a mathematical abstraction: an irrational number and an infinite decimal.

Simultaneously, however, when the man's limbs are arranged like a "T," he fits perfectly within a square. Squares are more "down to earth" than circles are—they're straightforward and built of right angles and rational numbers. They're easier to measure and understand. If circles are divine, squares are mortal. You'll notice, however, that he has a different center point in this arrangement: it's the base of the penis. This might give you a chuckle as you ponder the cosmic significance of genitalia, but I suppose it's safe to say that much of our mortal experience is grounded in this most human aspect of our being—and the biological trigger for the creation of life.

STRUCTURAL INTEGRITY IN PRACTICE

So, what does that overlap look like? What does it look like when we acknowledge our dual nature—body and soul—and do our best to live so that the two are integrated?

Let's imagine a high school senior named Evan. He's a hockey player and devoted athlete, and he is a pretty integrated young guy.

He trains hard, eats right, gets enough sleep, and avoids harmful habits like smoking and drinking. That's his body.

He has an emotional connection to hockey and all the relationships it involves, from his teammates and coaches to his friends and family. That's his heart.

He's committed to school, because he considers himself a scholar-athlete. He also studies technique and strategy related to hockey. That's his mind.

Likewise, he sees his athletic discipline as a spiritual undertaking—in fact, for Evan, the hard work is a sort of prayer and devotion to God. He prays regularly for guidance, patience, and stamina. That's his soul.

Evan lives in both the square and the circle, so to speak.

Now let's take a look at Alex. He's a classmate of Evan's, and he's on the same hockey team, but his life isn't as integrated. He also trains hard, maintains a healthy diet, and avoids harmful habits. His body is all-in.

He's a straight-A student, and that's because of his hard work and devotion to school. His mind is active and engaged.

The problem with Alex is that his "heart isn't in it," as they say—and neither is his soul. He doesn't take any joy in playing hockey or learning in school, and he doesn't invest in building relationships. He doesn't see the need to connect his heart and soul to his mind and body. As a result, his life feels imbalanced and "dis-integrated."

When Evan and Alex are confronted with the same challenge or obstacle, they might respond very differently. Let's say they are both taking a difficult, high-stakes test, and their eligibility to gain a scholarship to a top-tier hockey school is on the line. Each is presented with an opportunity to cheat, and the temptation is powerful.

For Alex, this is mostly a matter of the mind. He's focused on his odds of getting caught. He doesn't connect the decision to his heart or soul. He's far more likely to cheat. For Alex, there's no divine math involved—it's all right angles and easy equations.

Evan, however, feels the powerful influence of his heart and soul. While his mind can also calculate the chances of getting caught, he is focused more on his values and his conscience—not to mention how cheating would affect his relationships with his teammates, coaches, and parents. The stuff that's harder to measure. The math of virtues.

What does this mean for you?

I think making a good path involves the hard work of integrating these four aspects of our lives, reconciling the circle and the square. It's not easy. But you can use them as a sort of guide when you confront a difficult challenge or temptation. Ask yourself four questions of integrity:

- What is my *body* telling me?
- What is my *mind* telling me?
- What is my *heart* telling me?
- What is my *soul* telling me?

You can see how asking *all four* questions is powerful. Depending on the nature of the challenge or temptation, one or two of them might not be sufficient to help you maintain your moral integrity.

Let's say the temptation is to cheat on a test—which might seem mentally strategic—your mind might justify doing it. Your heart and soul will protest, though.

If the temptation is sexual, your body is probably not going to be too helpful, and your mind might not be too focused in that moment. You're all square in that moment, and remember where the center of the square is located. The circle of heart and soul may need to come to your rescue.

Sometimes, in a spiritual or emotional struggle, you might be confused as to what your heart and soul are telling you. Too circular. Too hard to nail down. In that case, maybe you need rely on your mind and your physical senses—lean into the square, if you will—to make a rational decision.

Imbalance, Excess, and Toxicity

Before I became an EMT, I was leading a group of students on a multiday backpacking trip in Utah's Zion National Park with another teacher. One of the boys began to feel weak and a little bit dizzy.

Given the rigorous climb in hot, dry, sunny weather, I assumed he was dehydrated and encouraged him to keep drinking, a little at a time. He agreed and emptied his water bottle over the course of the next mile, but he wasn't getting any better. One of his friends gave him another bottle of water. Surely, he must be dehydrated, we figured.

Except soon, he felt even worse. He was unsteady on his feet, and he even seemed a little confused. Now we were worried. As the other teacher and I discussed turning around, he sat with his friends, who were trying to keep his spirits up. One of them broke out a bag of trail mix, and they convinced him to eat a few handfuls of the sweet-and-salty blend of peanuts, chocolate, and raisins.

Ten minutes later, he felt fine. "Guess I just needed to eat," he said through a mouthful. "Skipped breakfast."

We kept an eye on him over the next few hours, but he was totally back to normal. His recovery had been rapid, like flipping a switch.

A year later, during EMT training, we were learning about blood chemistry and hydration. That's when I realized what had happened in Utah. My student hadn't been dehydrated at all.

It was essentially the opposite—he was hyponatremic. The sodium level in his blood had dipped dangerously low due to the heavy sweating and his failure to eat breakfast that morning. By encouraging him to drink more water, we were *hyperhydrating* him, which only made the hyponatremia worse as he continued to sweat out the little remaining sodium in his blood. When he ate the sugary, salty trail mix, his body adjusted rapidly.

When I described the situation to my EMT instructor, he mentioned another term for what the kid was experiencing: "water toxicity."

I tell you this story to make a point: anything can become toxic in excess. This is obvious when it comes to something like alcohol. But toxicity is possible, even from something that seems harmless by itself, like water.

The same applies to qualities, attitudes, and behaviors. If there's an aspect of our life that begins to become excessive, it can become toxic. Ambition at moderate levels is fine. Victor Frankenstein developed "toxic ambition."

CAN MASCULINITY ITSELF BE TOXIC?

You've probably heard of the term "toxic masculinity." It started showing up a lot in the late 2010s amid the #MeToo movement. I don't like it, because I think it's reductive and divisive.

There's nothing *inherently* wrong with masculinity, and the term makes it seem as though just by being a guy, you're potentially dangerous, and more so than if you're not a guy. (I don't think "toxic femininity" would be too popular, right?) When a term is so instantly polarizing, it tends to get in the way of its own meaning—because people roll their eyes and stop listening.

But let's give the devil his due. If you're old enough to be reading this book, you probably understand what "toxic masculinity" refers to—whether you like the term or not: It's when traditionally masculine traits and qualities become excessive, to the point of causing harm. What are "traditionally masculine" traits? Trying to define masculinity is tricky. It's sure to incite some strong feelings. Politics and philosophy aside, there are varied scientific opinions about the relationship between gender and biological sex.

I believe masculinity comes from a combination of nature (the way we're wired biologically) and nurture (the way our culture shapes us). They both matter. As for the biological component, research shows meaningful differences in how biologically male and female brains are wired. For example, brain scans have proven that when given the same task or asked the same question, there are consistent differences in which parts of male and female brains light up.[1] So there is a clear biological component.

Of course, the way we are raised and our cultural norms also influence what we consider masculine and feminine. Because I'm not a neuroscientist, I don't have an expert scientific opinion about the nature/nurture breakdown—that is, the degree to which masculine qualities come from being biologically male, and how much they come from what our culture teaches boys. But I think it's unwise to downplay biological sex differences. Despite the insistence of a small group of ideologically driven people who deny this, there *are* masculine qualities and tendencies that present overwhelmingly in males, and I've observed them for more than twenty-five years of working directly with boys and young men.

Some of the most compelling research I've encountered in this area comes from Michael Gurian, an author, therapist, and educator who has for the better part of forty years explored brain difference and the neuroscience behind it. It is worth noting that a February 2024 study by Stanford researchers, which was recently published in the *Proceedings of the National Academy of Sciences*, further supports the reality of sex-based brain differences that Gurian's work has explored for years.[2] This is far from a complete list, but here are some of Gurian's observations about sex-based tendencies, which are largely paraphrased from his book *The Wonder of Boys*, originally published in 1996 and updated in 2006:[3]

- **Nonverbal emotional expression:** Most men tend not to talk through their feelings; rather, they express them physically.
- **Task-solution orientation:** Most guys would rather get right to work fixing a problem than discuss it.

- **Spatial/kinesthetic orientation:** Guys tend to think visually and geometrically, and prefer active learning through hands-on experience.

- **Independence:** Most guys tend to want to solve their own problems rather than ask for help.

- **Aggressiveness and competitiveness:** Most guys tend to be competitive and become fairly aggressive in a competitive situation.

- **Assertiveness:** Most guys are quick to express their opinion and go after something they want.

Obviously, these are generalizations. As Gurian explains, there are outliers. Some men don't fit one or more of these at all; likewise, there are women who don't, either. For example, while most men are more assertive and aggressive than most women, there is a small minority of women who are more assertive and aggressive than most men. And, what's more, these traits overlap more than they don't, which is to say that men and women have much more in common than not. But the differences are there on average, and they matter. I bet if you think about the boys and men you know, compared to the girls and women you know, you'll agree these tendencies Gurian names are generally true.

An excess of any of these traits could be harmful to a guy himself. If you're so independent that you won't ask for help, that's not going to go well. If you're so averse to talking through your feelings that you never do, you're going to bottle things up until you explode. If you're so focused on fixing problems that you don't take time to really understand them, you're of limited use when it comes to preventing them from happening again. If you're so averse to reading and learning through discussion that you decide books and school just aren't for you, you're really limiting yourself.

Sure, these are all problems. But when people use the term "toxic masculinity," they're usually referring to either harmful attitudes or bad behaviors, but most often a combination of the two, because it's hard to separate attitudes from the behaviors they drive. Sometimes the harmful attitudes are obvious. We see them, for example, in the misogynist and the homophobe. As for the bad behaviors, they can certainly come from such harmful attitudes—and that's pretty obvious, especially when we hear young men parroting ignorant, disrespectful nonsense being spewed out by some of the less refined voices of the online "manosphere." But I think it's often more subtle. I think plenty of guys who *aren't*, at their core, misogynistic or homophobic (to use the same examples) can still act out plenty of behaviors that fuel the notion of toxic masculinity. From what I can see, these behaviors usually stem from an excess of one or both of the last two typically masculine traits I mentioned earlier: aggressiveness/competitiveness and assertiveness.

It's not hard to understand how aggression and competition can become toxic when taken too far. You can imagine any number of scenarios there—but you probably don't have to imagine them. You've probably seen plenty of it. It's one thing to be a "physical player" on the lacrosse field. It's another to be that annoying guy who's hypercompetitive in every aspect of his life.

I think most of the "toxic masculinity" references have to do with an excess of assertiveness. Being assertive—that is, being confident and willing to express your opinions and stand up for yourself—is important. Being excessively assertive makes you an overbearing jerk who comes across as feeling entitled to whatever you want. I suppose it's fair to call that "toxic assertiveness."

Take this in a sexual context, though, and being too assertive can become a different kind of problem. A healthy amount of sexual expression is necessary in a healthy, consensual sexual relationship. But feeling entitled to make unwelcome sexual advances? That's a recipe for big trouble. I believe there are plenty of things in our culture that fuel the excesses that result in toxic sexual attitudes and behavior—a sort of "toxic hyper-sexuality." One of them is online pornography, and we'll talk about that in a later chapter.

Let's imagine two different guys again, to get a picture of what excess might look like compared to balance.

First, we see Rishi. He's a young investment banker in his early twenties, just out of college. He plays in a men's soccer league, and he's known for his high-energy, very physical presence on the field. He's vocal, forceful, and aggressive, and it gets him an occasional penalty. He has no shortage of wise-cracks among his teammates, and he's known to have a bit of a mouth when he's "in the zone" while playing—hence those penalties. But Rishi draws a clear line between his behaviors on and off the soccer field. When it comes to his professional demeanor, he's respectful and never uses vulgarity. He keeps his trademark humor in check at work, and he avoids saying things that he knows might make others uncomfortable. On the dating scene, Rishi keeps his sexuality in check, too—he's not afraid to be physical, but he doesn't make assumptions and he communicates clearly to ensure there's consent. He also reins in his sexual behavior in keeping with the teachings of his family and his religious traditions—these are all forces that help him maintain appropriate boundaries and limits. He integrates his body, mind, soul, and heart, like we discussed previously.

Dan is a different story. Dan works with Rishi, and he plays on the same men's soccer club team. Dan's not as physically imposing as Rishi, but he's quick, and likewise an aggressive, physical player who gets noticed on the field. Dan's also a notorious fountain of off-color humor in the locker room, frequently spouting the kind of sexually charged jokes that raise eyebrows even among his often-raucous teammates. The real difference between Dan and Rishi comes when they leave the soccer club, though. Dan seems to exert the same outward force everywhere, including the office. He doesn't filter his comments or humor there, and he makes people uncomfortable with things he says. When it comes to his social interactions, Dan's presumptuous and forward both with friends and strangers. He likes to assert his strength by being curt and rude to waitstaff at restaurants. He sees the dating scene as a game of dominance and strategy, with little interest in building any lasting relationships. In fact, he seems interested more in racking up stories of sexual conquest that he can share indiscriminately, whether in the locker room or in the office.

Both of these young men exhibit the typical masculine qualities and tendencies I mentioned earlier, none of which is inherently bad to begin with. In fact, at healthy, balanced levels, they are quite important for a functioning society—and in some cases, desirable leadership attributes. But while Rishi seems to maintain that balance, Dan lets things go out of balance. It's when these qualities hit levels of excess like this that they cause harm to oneself or others. And yes, it's fair to call that "toxic." But I still don't like the term "toxic masculinity." I think society could have a more productive conversation using words that are easier to understand without being so immediately divisive. Maybe something simpler, like "unbalanced" or just "unhealthy."

Our Heroes Are Integrated

The *Vitruvian Man* shows us structural integrity.

That kind of integrity embodies the characteristics we admire in the men we call heroes: men who strive to embrace the truth, stand up for what's right, treat others with respect, make personal sacrifices for the greater good, defend the vulnerable, and work hard—whether or not anyone is looking.

That's a man of integrity—an integrated man.

That's the kind of man who strives to make a good path.

That's the kind of man who can be someone's hero.

You can be that guy.

CHAPTER TEN

Traveling Companions

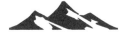

CONSIDER THIS STORY. A guy in his twenties named Eric takes an autumn hike alone in a remote area. He's in good shape and pretty experienced. It's just a day hike, and he's done it before, so he doesn't go overboard with his gear beyond the basics. Comfortable and familiar with the trail, he gets a later start than he usually would, and he lingers a little longer on the scenic ridge.

By the time Eric starts his descent, it's mid-afternoon. This time of year, the light starts to fade by early evening. Realizing that he'll be late meeting his buddies to watch a game later on, he picks up the pace.

The weather changes rapidly, as it often does in the mountains. The temperature drops, and before long, the mild conditions become windy, with rain slashing at his face. Within minutes, the temperature plummets. The rain turns into freezing rain, and finally to driving snow. Rocks and tree roots have just enough time to get soaked before the mercury dips sufficiently low to form a thin, shimmering layer of ice.

And that's when Eric slips, howling with pain as his ankle twists the wrong way. As he falls, the momentum of his backpack is just enough to knock him further off balance, and half a second later, he's half-sliding, half-rolling down a steep ravine, unable to stop.

After what seems like a full minute of uncontrolled flailing, Eric blinks up to see he's fallen at least eighty or ninety feet down into a streambed, and he feels the icy water soaking his boots and clothes. He scrambles out of the water, shivering, his ankle pulsing with white-hot pain. When he reaches for his backpack to find the emergency kit with his matches, fire starters, and flashlight, he realizes it must have flown off of him during the fall. He can't find it, and it's getting dark.

When he tries to walk, his ankle buckles, and he screams in agony. It's broken. Less than an hour later, he's deeply hypothermic, past the point of shivering and unable to think clearly.

It isn't long before he decides to take just a little rest.

He doesn't feel too cold anymore as he fades.

***

This is not a true story. It's based on a case study that I designed during the wilderness search and rescue portion of EMT school. I'm retelling it here because it shows the danger of walking a difficult path alone.

The slip was not Eric's mistake. That was an accident.

His mistake was traveling alone.

And because of that, Eric died of a broken ankle.

The Gift of Friendship

I got to know my friend Scott in high school, long before he became the best man at my wedding. We were classmates and teammates in both crew and swimming. We're physical opposites—I'm short and stocky; he's tall and lean. Other than that, we have a lot in common. We share a lot of values. We have similar taste in movies, literature, and music.

Our friendship took root in these shared experiences and characteristics, of course, but the key to our lasting bond is the fact that we are equally happy being busy together or doing nothing together.

When many of our other friends were out doing more exciting things on Friday nights, we were usually content just to drive around and talk or watch a movie. Since we often had practice at dawn, our evenings were pretty tame.

We had some adventures, including a long-weekend road trip in the summer before our senior year. One of our favorite things to do was crack open a road atlas and plan the ultimate cross-country road trip we'd take someday.

When I headed to the Coast Guard Academy, Scott headed to the Naval Academy at Annapolis. You know my story—but Scott stayed with it and remained in the service for more than a decade. Meanwhile, I did take a cross-country road trip with a mutual friend of ours, but Scott was on a ship somewhere.

He got married a few years before I did. His wife was also a Navy officer, and she was deployed shortly after their wedding. It was the middle of the summer, and Scott found himself alone on an extended leave without much to do. I was living the life of a bachelor teacher: single, with the summer off. Scott called me up to see if I wanted to get together for a beer. I suggested we do one better and take that road trip.

So, we did. Just like that.

We got in my Jeep and left the following day. We drove more than three thousand miles to the west coast, with a circuitous route that took us into the Rockies and across the deserts of Arizona, Utah, and New Mexico. We met up with my brother for a while; we also picked up another buddy who traveled with us for part of the trip. It was a journey full of adventure, and I have vivid memories of the spectacular grandeur of the mountains, deserts, sky, stars, rivers, lakes, and the Pacific Ocean. We talked for hours about everything under the sun. We'd laugh, agree, and sometimes disagree. He'd often drive too fast. I'd sometimes drive too slow. But no matter what, we'd always agree to disagree and keep smiling. But just as vivid are my memories of the long stretches of comfortable quiet as we drove across the vast landscape, listening to music or just the sound of the tires on the road. Often, hours would pass without a word between us. We could just *be*, and silence never felt awkward.

That trip is symbolic of our friendship in many ways, but I think it's also symbolic of genuine companionship—the kind of bond between and among people who find as much joy in shared, spontaneous adventure as with each other's simple presence.

Our Need for Companionship

Humans aren't wired to live alone. We thrive in communities. Across the millennia and across cultures, families and communities form the gravitational centers of human life. It's a matter of survival—there's strength in numbers. In fact, if you leave one of us in isolation for long enough, we'll go crazy. Don't get me wrong—we all need solitude—but there's a difference between solitude and isolation.

Solitude is a peaceful state of mind that allows us time to reflect, discern, and enjoy a respite from all the noise of the world. Solitude is a retreat from everyone else, but not an escape from them; a retreat that allows us inward focus to more fully re-invest ourselves in the world.

Isolation, on the other hand, is a way of escape that turns in on us; as we turn away from the world—as we avoid it and other people—we lose not just them, but ourselves. We aren't wired for isolation. Having true companions empowers us to enjoy solitude without being plunged into the loneliness that comes with isolation.

Sociologists, psychologists, and medical professionals have increasingly made clear the "crisis of friendship" experienced by men. Perhaps the starkest indication that men are suffering from isolation lies in data from the National Institutes of Mental

Health, which tell us the suicide rate was four times higher for men than it was for women in 2020.[1]

A lot of guys are lonely at the core—especially as they get older. That's one of the ironies: While many of us build close-knit "bands of brothers" during childhood and adolescence, those bands tend to fade as we grow into adulthood. It's easy to understand why. Our culture is full of structures that facilitate friendship when we're young. We're on teams together, we're in clubs together, we're in school together. Put simply, we grow up together. But when the growing up part is more or less behind us—when we are required to set forth on our own paths—the going can get very rough indeed. For many men, the cruel irony is that the vital intensity of the strong boyhood friendships they remember makes their loneliness as adults all the more painful.

And yet, traveling companions are vital as we make our path. We need older, wiser ones to guide us. We need peers to travel alongside us. Eventually, we might discover the joy that lies in serving as experienced guides for younger companions who follow us.

"Companion" derives from Latin, meaning "a person with whom one breaks bread." This is to share one of the most basic, essential human experiences—eating together. Different cultures all over the world have variations on the same tendency to gather with others around food, whether at the table or on the ground. We bolster strength and build the "self" we are creating as we grow up by sharing food with our companions.

Some of the strength and growing self comes from table fellowship, the opportunity to communicate deeply as we share joys and sorrows. It is no coincidence that the major world religions center many of their most important rituals around a table, and very often key elements involve food—consuming it, abstaining from it, engaging in fasts. Secular holidays like Thanksgiving do the same.

We get to know each other around tables. We are reminded of our humanity when we break bread with others. This most basic of foods we consume as humans draws from wheat, a plant that takes root in the *humus*, the earth.

You might say that everyone with whom we develop a meaningful relationship is a companion. But if you reflect upon the many people who have accompanied you at various times in your life, relatively few have had the most powerful and meaningful connection.

There is value in taking some time to identify and recognize this group of people. This gives you a chance to consider the value of your most important relationships and whether you have been investing in them accordingly. One of the most important investments in any relationship is gratitude—and sometimes we just don't express it enough. Eric, the hiker from the case study, would have been very grateful in his ravine for just one of these companions by his side.

Who is the person you would want with you, whether during a challenging adventure or a long road trip? Take a moment to think about that person, and call to mind gratitude. Do you think they know you feel this way? Have you expressed your gratitude lately?

Risking Emotional Connection

If you ever have a little kid, you will probably find yourself saying "Use your words!" This is what we say to frustrated toddlers who are throwing a tantrum. As the father of two sons and a daughter, I have already seen a difference between them: I have to remind my boys to use their words more often.

I don't think that pattern changes as we get older. For a lot of guys, it's one thing to *show* people how we feel, but another entirely to *tell* them. The latter takes a little more openness. As a guy, you've probably noticed that boys and men tend to bond and connect by facing something together—we see this in our sports and games. We see this when we build something together or do yardwork together. Sometimes this involves conversation; often it doesn't. Doing something together is a form of bonding, for sure.

But we could benefit from more direct conversation, too.

Let's consider the risk we take when we make ourselves vulnerable through openness. The conventional wisdom about men is that we don't express our feelings, or that maybe we don't even have them! You know this second part is nonsense. Of course we have feelings. The first part, about emotional expression, has something to it, though. Communication comes in many forms, both verbal and nonverbal.

Back in chapter 9, "The Integrated Man," I referred to typical trait differences between men and women. This is one of them. Generally speaking, women are far more inclined to engage in verbal emotional expression—talking through their feelings—than men are. As you probably know, guys often tend to use nonverbal communication to express emotion.

As one of five brothers and the product of an all-boys' school—not to mention having worked with young guys for a lot of years—I understand how a not-so-gentle punch to the shoulder, coupled with a smile, can be a show of affection. Maybe you do, too. The high-fives, chest-bumps, and affectionate roughhousing among teammates are all examples of typically male, nonverbal emotional expression.

In my experience, girls and women sometimes don't recognize the emotional weight of boys' and men's nonverbal communication, and instead resentfully believe they're getting the "silent treatment." But sometimes this is what it looks like when boys and men are saying plenty—just not using words. And while I do think it would be helpful for more girls and women to recognize the nonverbal expression offered by boys and men, I think there's much more work to be done *by* boys and men when it comes to communicating.

Sorry, guys, but we have to work on this.

Most guys feel about as comfortable talking about feelings as they do sitting in the dentist's chair. Our culture has done well to convince us that a guy giving credence to emotional vulnerability is tantamount to not only *admitting* weakness, but also succumbing to it.

Obviously, that's not true. Being emotional and being tough are not mutually exclusive. If a guy's "toughness" is threatened by something as natural as expressing his emotions, it's not very tough, is it?

Nonetheless, if we do share personal things with our companions, including genuine emotional expressions, there is a degree of vulnerability that we've agreed to. That does carry risks. If I tell you about some ways in which I'm a mess, you have dirt on me. You could use it against me. That's true. It's a risk. It's also one worth taking, judiciously.

Scott has plenty of dirt on me. But I'm glad he does.

I'm not suggesting we should share every feeling we have. That's ridiculous. I am saying it's worth being open and honest and taking the risk of self-disclosure, because the alternative is a life of emotional isolation and the pain of repressed, bottled-up feelings—not to mention fears and anxieties that we never share. Those feelings have to go somewhere, and they'll probably end up coming out anyway—in some more explosive, or at least harmful, manner.

There are some strategies you can use if you want to have more conversations. First, if you're not comfortable just sitting and talking face to face, then don't just sit and talk face to face. There's no reason you can't have deep conversation *while* you're going for a walk, tossing a ball back and forth, driving, or tackling some chore together. When I'm trying to have a deep conversation with a male friend, male colleague, or one of the guys I teach, I always try to build in some movement.

This doesn't mean you shouldn't ever strive to make eye contact and talk face to face. But I wouldn't use that as the main measure of the quality of a conversation.

You'll also find that the more you practice articulating your feelings, the easier and less awkward it gets. It's a hell of a thing to talk about your fears. They tend to diminish when you do. It's like opening the window shades, letting sunlight into a darkened room.

Ironically, a good starting place for sharing your emotions might be with a group of people who *aren't* your best friends. In some ways, that's the power of the retreat-style experiences I mentioned in the chapter on pilgrimage. Sometimes it's easier to open up with people when you've intentionally wandered beyond the scope of your daily routines. This can take several forms. It could be as simple as joining a casual sports league—for example, playing soccer or basketball at a local park. Or joining a running group, or meeting a regular group to work out at a gym. Or even joining a book club.

Maybe, however, you just want to get right to the point, and be part of a group specifically built for opening up. Many guys, for example, join men's support groups just for this purpose—to open up, to be vulnerable, and to relate to each other through shared activity and intentional conversation. If you're not sure how to break the ice and be more open with your own circle of family and friends, maybe consider exploring something along those lines. It can be a starting point. The simple fact that so many such organizations and programs for men exist is all the proof you need: you're not the only guy out there seeking emotional connection and meaningful bonds.

There are risks in being open with your emotions and talking with your companions about personal things. Pains. Fears. Struggles. Failures. Successes. Challenges. Hopes. Joys. Aspirations. There are risks, but I think the risks are higher if we *don't* become open about these things with others.

TRUE BROTHERHOOD

Since this is a book written for young guys, it is worth putting some focus now on brotherhood. Having coached and taught at boys' prep schools for so long, I have very often heard references to the powerful "brotherhood" that exists at schools or among teammates. I'm one of five brothers, and I believe powerfully in the notion of brotherhood in the metaphoric sense: a powerful bond that links hearts together. Indeed, I think it's very important for a boy or man to be part of a "band of brothers."

(By the way, this doesn't have to be exclusively male—in reality, this is probably a "band of brothers and sisters." With that said, I think all-male spaces have an important role to play for men, just as I think all-female spaces do for women. In any case, I'm going to stick with "brotherhood" to make my point.)

If you know anything about boys, you know that brotherhood is very much about loyalty. About having one another's back. That's good stuff. Except, here's the thing: true brothers understand that having one another's back also means holding each other accountable—and sometimes that means doing something very difficult. That might mean telling your brother something he doesn't want to hear but needs to hear. Sometimes it might even mean forcing him to face consequences.

We all know the old adage that "snitches get stitches." But sometimes the stitches are worth it, if the snitching is necessary to keep your brother from going down a seriously bad path. True loyalty isn't about blind allegiance. It isn't about covering up bad behavior. It isn't about keeping your brother free from consequences. In fact, that's not brotherhood at all. That's setting him up for a bigger fall later on.

Let's say you have a buddy who's getting into a behavior or habit that's bad news, like experimenting with drugs, acting inappropriately with girls, or repeatedly cheating in school. You want to call him out on it, but he's your friend, and you want to be loyal, and after all, snitches get stitches. You don't want to rock the boat. Totally understandable.

Here's the problem, though. By avoiding short-term tension between the two of you, you might be setting him up for a far more painful situation later. Genuine loyalty sometimes means we have to risk our brothers getting pretty ticked off at us. That's part of the cost of *true* loyalty. You can't call it true loyalty if it requires you to betray your core values. Loyalty to a friend, even as he pursues something that runs contrary to virtue, isn't really loyalty in its truest form. Genuine loyalty would mean doing what's required to help him be his *best* self, in pursuit of his *genuine* desires. If you know him well enough to call him your brother, you must know that those genuine desires don't include doing things that are self-destructive.

They call it "turning a blind eye" for a reason. Brothers shouldn't be blind toward one another. That isn't real companionship. When it comes to holding each other accountable, it's better to face a short-term consequence in the interest of the long-term relationship than the alternative. *Truly* having each other's back sometimes feels like betrayal in the short term. If it's a genuine brotherhood, though, it will endure that discomfort once the dust settles.

If your friends—especially the ones you'd call your brothers—don't hold you accountable and vice versa, maybe it's time to re-evaluate those relationships. At the same time, you might consider this question: What people truly hold me to account because they genuinely want to help me move toward my telos? Those are your true friends. Those are your real brothers and sisters.

―――

While parts of our personal pilgrimage can and should be traveled in solitude, the quest for moral excellence is not meant to be undertaken alone.

It's vital to develop meaningful companionship, and that takes work. Take time to reflect upon your relationships with your friends. Ascertain who is a true companion to you, and to whom you're a true companion.

Be sure to express gratitude—and do it shamelessly, openly. Use your words. Tell people you love them, and be clear about it.

Yeah, it might feel awkward. It's worth the sidelong glances.

And if you find that the sort of honest, genuine connection of companionship is lacking or absent in your life, you'll want to put some work in. That might mean taking some risks and opening up. It might mean putting yourself out there and trying new things. Find that band of brothers and sisters and hang on to them. Solitude is healthy and important, but isolation—well, that can really get heavy after a while.

Traveling alone for too long is dangerous.

CHAPTER ELEVEN

Machine Maintenance

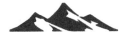

As I MENTIONED in an earlier chapter, my paternal grandfather died of a heart attack, back when my dad was fifteen. Obviously, my mother, brothers, and I never got to meet him. He was only forty-two, which is a few years younger than I am now. There were a lot of things working against him. For one thing, he was a smoker, long before there was widespread understanding of how harmful it was. Then there was just a little bit of stress, I'm sure, from his Army service during World War II, both in Europe and the Pacific. Nonetheless, he wasn't overweight—from what I can tell from the pictures I've seen, he was slimmer than I am, by a good margin. Whatever the reason, the main point is he died when my dad was fifteen, leaving him at a time when a boy really needs his father.

Don't get me wrong—I'm not *blaming* the man. Who am I to judge someone I've never met, who lived through circumstances I've never known? But it's fair to conclude that he didn't live as long as he might have with some better preventive maintenance—that is, better self-care. Ultimately, he didn't get to be a companion to his wife or son for very long. He never got to be a companion to his five grandsons or twelve great-grandchildren. His path was good, but it was short.

I don't want that to happen to my wife and kids. That's why I take the cholesterol medication I'm on, why I've begun to get serious about keeping an eye on what I eat, why I exercise at least a little bit every day, and why I now make sure to see my primary physician and dentist regularly.

We don't live that long.

Seriously, man. We don't. That fact hits like a wave that knocks you over when you realize you're statistically closer to death than birth. At least it did for me. That was right about the same time I started to experience things like plantar fasciitis, significant hair loss, and a host of other relatively minor maladies that find their way into our lives as we age.

Chances are, since you're reading a book intended for boys and young men, you're probably nowhere near your forties, so all of this may seem fairly distant and irrelevant. If you're a young guy in good health, it seems counterintuitive to do a lot of preventive maintenance.

But that's sort of like saying that just because your car runs fine now, there's really no need to fuss over things like regular oil changes, fluid checks, tire rotations, filter replacements, or brake pad inspections.

Trust me, pal. Getting old is coming for you.

Look, it's not a bad thing. After all, as my very wise grandmother has often said with a good-natured chuckle, getting older is much better than the alternative.

So don't be afraid of aging. Just be smart, stay humble, and take care of yourself.

THE TWO FOUNDATIONS

There's a great parable in the Gospel of Matthew called "The Two Foundations." It lays out the prospect of two builders—a wise one who builds on a foundation of rock, and a foolish one who builds on a foundation of sand. When the storms and heavy rains come, the house built on a poor foundation is washed away.

Similarly, if you don't make the efforts to take care of yourself, you won't have the strength to face life's proverbial storms ourselves. You certainly won't be able to help others weather their storms, either. Adequate self-care, then, is a matter of both wisdom and humility—but it's also just practical.

MACHINE COMPONENTS

Back in the chapter called "The Integrated Man," we discussed the importance of connecting the four components of our body, mind, heart, and soul. But you also need to keep *each* of these in good shape to make and travel a good path.

This book is full of advice for taking care of your mind, heart, and soul. This chapter focuses a little bit more on the body, with a bit of the heart involved, too. The square part, if you will, of the dual nature depicted in the illustration of the *Vitruvian Man*. You know I'm not a doctor, so this is not a chapter about medical advice. It's a few thoughts based on what I picked up as an EMT and years of coaching and mentoring young guys. You've got to keep up preventive maintenance of the machine that has the privilege of housing your soul for the time being.

Maintaining the Body

By this age, you've heard plenty about what *not* to do. I could put together a long list like that, but you've probably already heard all that. Let's focus instead on stuff you *should* do. After all, "preventive maintenance" involves the verb *maintain*, which implies taking action. Here are seven things I suggest you do:

1. Get more sleep.

2. Hydrate better.

3. Brush and floss better.

4. Exercise and stretch a little every day.

5. Take care of your eyes and your neck.

6. Change your sheets.

7. Build a doctor-patient relationship.

Get more sleep. The American Academy of Pediatrics says teenagers should get eight to ten hours of sleep. If you're getting up at six, you really should be hitting the rack by ten, at least while you're a teenager. Most guys I've taught over the years have reported staying up much later than that—usually looking at screens, which only compounds the problem, given how addicting those can be. You know how different you feel after a good night's rest—especially if you don't normally get enough.

Back in EMT school, we learned that most people are suboptimally hydrated at any given moment. That doesn't mean we're all chronically dehydrated and should be hauling around ridiculously big water bottles on a regular day at school or the office, but it does mean most of us would probably be better off drinking a little more water. The instructor explained that even minor levels of dehydration can reduce the efficiency of all sorts of physiological systems—things like autoimmune functions, tissue recovery after injury, metabolism, concentration, and mood regulation. If you're well hydrated, you're probably going to have a more stable blood sugar level that's less likely to spike and crash. It also tends to help control your appetite. If you're like me and you'd like to lose a few pounds, drink more water—especially just before you're going to eat.

Brush and floss better. Yeah, I know. Sounds basic. Dentists will tell you, though, that most of us don't floss as often as we should, and most of us don't brush properly. Do you do it the right way? For as long as they advise? Along the gumline? If you feel like it'd be too silly to ask if you're doing it wrong, well, get over it. Something you do twice a day, every day, for your entire life is probably worth getting right . . . right? I wish I could say honestly that I floss my teeth every day. I'm working on it. Life is hard.

A little bit of exercise every day goes a long way. This is one of those areas where I think it's easy to underestimate the importance of consistency and the value of even moderate investment.

Remember Will Durant's paraphrase of Aristotle? "We are what we repeatedly do." This obviously goes for exercise.

We encourage ourselves when we hold ourselves to meaningful routines. There's as much value in the disciplined habit as there is in the exercise itself. Sure, the physical benefit is clear—you don't need a medical degree to know that. But it's reaffirming to know that you're capable of sticking to something, even if it's relatively light and simple.

A lot of guys are athletes and have good training when it comes to fitness and strength development. Even if you're not, doing the most basic things is so, so much better than doing nothing at all. If all you do is go for a brisk twenty-minute walk every day, you are way ahead of the curve.

From what I've seen, the best sustainable impact seems to come from combining cardio work with weight training. It doesn't have to be complicated. You don't need expert knowledge to do basic strength training exercises. You don't need a weight room, either. Learn some basic routines, even using nothing more than bodyweight resistance movements if you want, and stick to it. When it comes to exercise, even a little bit, done consistently, is infinitely better than nothing at all.

Stretching a little bit every day will keep you feeling better and help you avoid injury. If you don't know how to stretch, look it up online. On the days when I can't find the time or energy to work out, I try, at the very least, to stretch for a few minutes—even if it's while I'm doing something else, like looking at my phone or reading. Again, like the exercise bit—doing just a little bit is so much better than none at all, as long as you're doing it properly.

Take care of your eyes and neck. This is something I really didn't understand until middle age. It was only in my late thirties, after a solid decade and a half constantly looking at screens, I started to notice my eyesight changing. Part of this is no doubt simply a matter of age. But with the hours and hours of screen time, I've found that my eyes get dry and irritated much more often than they ever used to. I've also noticed myself becoming increasingly nearsighted. Apparently, experts have seen this happening to us on a broad level, and at younger ages than ever before.[1] Some eye care professionals recommend a good practice is to take a break from looking at screens every twenty minutes or so, focusing on something about twenty feet away for at least twenty seconds. This might help stave off eye strain and maybe even (over the long term) myopia. Since your generation has been glued to screens from a much younger age than mine, I imagine you might be dealing with this even earlier. Maybe you already are.

Speaking of screen-related issues, take care of your neck. No doubt you've heard of "tech-neck." If you're like me, all those hours staring at screens with your neck craned down can take a toll. I realized how stiff my neck had become when I went to do a recent painting job that involved craning my neck to look *up* for an extended period. I was sore for days! If you look down at your phone or tablet for hours and have a stiff neck as a young man, be aware that it's not going to get better as you get older—it gets worse. Stretch and move accordingly. As I tried to work the knots out of my stiff neck muscles recently, it occurred to me that maybe if I looked up at the heavens as often as I looked down at my phone, I wouldn't have this problem. I chuckled at the thought, because I'm sure there's a deeper meaning there.

Change your sheets—and do all the other little things that most guys tend to neglect. This might apply more to you if you're older and living on your own in a bachelor pad, but even if you're still in high school you can get started. Clean the toilet from time to time. Get used to lifting the toilet seat to take a leak, if you don't already, and then always close the toilet lid before you flush. Following this simple advice will solve several problems at once. First, it will keep disgusting aerosolized fragments of human waste from pluming out of the toilet and onto your toothbrush every time you flush. Second, it will prevent the emergence of a new cold war between you and any current or future female companions who share your bathroom. Disregard this advice at your peril, but don't say you weren't warned.

Wipe down the germ-ridden surfaces of your phone, tablet, and keyboard from time to time. They are really gross. Clean that gunk out of year ears, for God's sake. Maybe you don't notice it, but other people sure do. How often do you change your sheets? You sweat a lot every night. You shed lots of skin cells every night. There's a good chance you drool on your pillowcase every night. Oil excretions from your pores make their way onto your pillow at night. Perhaps there are occasional other emissions. That's a lot of stuff accumulating on the sheets you're sleeping in, amigo. Most guys don't change their sheets often enough.

As the old saying goes, you can lead a horse to water, but you cannot make him drink. When I say "build a doctor-patient relationship," I'm talking about developing a meaningful working relationship with a range of people—a primary care physician, a dentist, and maybe others, such as a psychologist or therapist. The *patient* has to make the effort to see the doctor. Not everyone has easy access to a doctor. There are obstacles to this for many people, depending on any number of circumstances. But for most people in the developed world, expert health care is accessible.

Assuming that it is accessible, though, the effort piece is important. If you are fortunate enough to have a primary care physician, do you work at building that relationship? Do you make regular appointments, keep them, and then follow up on the advice and recommendations offered? Do you actually take prescribed medications as instructed? Do you have the where-withal and the humility to ask questions about your health, including awkward ones? I wonder how many people don't get care and treatment they should because they never bring themselves to explain or ask about an awkward, embarrassing, or uncomfortable situation.

This chapter is entitled "Machine Maintenance," and I really think that's the tack we have to take when it comes to speaking with our doctors about taking care of our bodies. We have to be willing to open up the hood and let the professionals take a close look at the engine—and we have to get over ourselves in order to do that. What's the alternative?

A Strategy for Handling Negative Emotions

Everything we just covered has to do with the physical body. But what about the heart? Just as you have to take care of the moving parts of the machine, you have to maintain your emotional health. Of course, entire books have been written about that, and I'll keep this to just a few thoughts about handling negative emotions. We've already looked at how guys struggle to express our emotions sometimes. Nonetheless, we both know that guys *have* plenty of deep, powerful emotions. The waters at the base of the Grand Canyon run deep.

I'll offer you one simple strategy for handling almost any negative emotion: gratitude.

I find that anytime I take a minute to muster some gratitude, in just about *any* situation, good will come of it, and I'll feel better, too. Gratitude has a way of putting things in perspective. It helps me focus on the graces and gifts present in my life. Consider how calling gratitude to mind can help with some negative emotions we all wrestle with.

Anger. Because anger is a quick emotion, it can take us by surprise. The people we love most can be the hardest to live with—but it's hard to stay angry with someone if you force yourself to reflect on your gratitude for that person.

Envy and jealousy. These are related, but not the same. If you want something someone else has—a quality, an attribute, or a possession—that's envy. When you envy the *relationship* a person has with someone other than you, that's jealousy. In either case, gratitude helps you focus on what you *do* have versus what you don't.

Sadness usually comes from loss or absence. It can range from just feeling down to powerful experiences of grief. How can gratitude help there? We can be grateful for what we *had*, even in the face of loss. Moreover, we can be grateful for what brings us joy—and that can help keep things in perspective.

Resentment. This is a particularly nasty emotion, because it creeps up on us. It's what happens when we slowly build a grudge about something—and very often, say nothing about it. Instead, we silently hold it over someone as it grows larger and larger. Eventually, something triggers us and the pent-up resentment comes flooding out in an explosion.

The worst thing about resentment is that we tend to build it into the relationships that matter most: our closest friends, our family members, or our spouse. Gratitude, therefore, is especially valuable here. It's like a pressure release valve that works against resentment. As tiny annoyances build up each day, we lower the pressure by recalling the gift of the people who annoy us. Of course, it doesn't hurt to address the sources of resentment *before* they build—and gratitude can help us do that lovingly.

Guilt and shame are nasty feelings. What does gratitude have to do with those? We often feel guilty or ashamed when we've wronged someone—sometimes without them even knowing it. Gratitude can help us rediscover our appreciation and respect for the person we've wronged—and it can encourage us to seek forgiveness, which we all need.

Obviously, mindful gratitude isn't the catch-all solution for handling every negative emotion. But it's a great starting place for making things better. Calling ourselves to gratitude forces us to slow down, think, and keep things in perspective.

It helps us maintain balance.

The Body Carries the Soul for a While

We're both circle and square. Our bodies are temporary. Like many people of faith, I believe that there's more to us than our bodies and that our souls live beyond the temporal form. But there's no reason not to take the best care possible of the amazing machine we embody for the duration.

We're also complex emotional beings, and taking care of our emotional health isn't optional. We need humility and wisdom to appreciate our human limitations and do the right maintenance. It's a survival skill. Without it, it's hard to get very far on whatever path we're traveling.

———

Back in the summer of 2011, I was on a school service learning trip with a group of students and teachers, living and working in El Faro, a remote mountain village in the Dominican Republic, for a good portion of the summer.

We were assisting the community with the construction of a road bridge across a sizable river. The lack of a bridge cut the small village off from neighboring towns whenever the river would swell from the frequent rains, making everyday life more difficult. Even more problematic were the frequent flash floods that had claimed several lives over the years. As we ate lunch with the workers one day, one of the men tearfully recalled the story of a mother and her two small children who had been killed while crossing just a few years back.

The construction plans called for five heavy cement piers spaced roughly twenty feet apart to complete the span. We hired an excavator to do the initial digging; everything after that was done by hand. Each pier took two full days of labor, and that was with about forty of us hauling, mixing, and pouring cement by hand. I don't recall the exact dimensions or the measure of concrete that went into each, but it was a lot. I mean, many, many tons, along with hundreds of basketball-sized boulders, which we passed along from man to man in a long chain from the creek bed.

By the end of each day, we were ragged, exhausted, soaked, and covered in cement. Talk about bonding. Within a few days, we were laughing and joking with our Dominican host families like old friends.

Near the end of the first week of work, just as we'd filled the scaffolding of the third pier with wet concrete, afternoon clouds gathered quickly and the sky grew dark. The locals began shouting for us to gather the tools and get out of the river. Everyone scrambled as the first lightning flashed across the sky and thunder rumbled. The Dominicans ushered us further up the hill, away from the banks. They pointed upriver and told us to watch.

At first, we heard a low rumble, which soon turned into a deafening roar. Seconds later, a furious torrent of muddy water rushed down the mountainside, carrying uprooted trees and massive boulders with it. It slammed into the bridge, demolishing the day's progress.

Later on, when the skies cleared, we surveyed the damage. Everyone was dismayed at the day's lost work. Our engineer lamented the loss of materials—thousands of dollars' worth of cement, rebar, and lumber had been washed away in seconds. Despite the massive weight of the still-unhardened cement and the immense boulders encased in iron rebar, it stood no chance against the river's fury.

But the first two piers were a different story. They contained the exact same materials, but the cement had cured already. Their foundations had set over the past week.

They withstood the flood with barely a scratch or a nick.

Your foundation will matter when tested. It takes time to build a strong one—and it takes some time for the cement to cure. So take care of yourself.

CHAPTER TWELVE

Service and Leadership

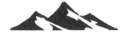

LUNCH STRIKES FEAR into the hearts of freshmen on the first day of high school. A lucky few arrive with a cadre from middle school. Many others have a reliable crew of teammates with whom they've already bonded in preseason summer workouts. They swagger to their chosen table as a pack, barely a break in their lively conversation as they dig in.

But some aren't so lucky. They don't know where to sit. They stand there, clutching a tray or brown bag lunch, eyes darting nervously in the desperate search. The next thirty minutes can be agonizing. Some make awkward attempts at conversation. Some don't bother and stake out a table alone. Never before have they longed for math class to begin; now, they count down the minutes.

That's why I found it so heartwarming some years back when a group of older guys at our school, instead of heading to the senior lounge, decided to fan out among the new freshmen and join them for lunch. These were the veterans—the top of the high school food chain. Among the group I counted two varsity team captains, the guy with the highest average in the senior class, the lead vocalist in a popular student band, and the student body president.

To freshmen, these guys might as well have been twenty-five. The facial hair and taller build alone put them in a different territory—the realm of men. But even immature sophomores can grow a scruffy beard. No, it was the seniors' easy confidence, friendly demeanor, and calm presence that marked them unmistakably as big brother figures.

As leaders.

Each one found a freshman sitting alone, chatted a bit, and then joined up with one or two others to form a table. It was like watching sheepdogs at work, corralling their flock.

Once gathered, they stayed with them long enough to smooth the awkward introductions and drum up some friendly conversation before dropping some fist bumps and taking off, leaving the group of newly introduced kids together.

This simple act of service cost these seniors practically nothing, other than a little time and energy. It wasn't a heavy lift, and no, they don't deserve medals for it. But they had nothing to gain, either. They just chose to lift someone up, and it meant the world to those freshmen, who from that day forward didn't sit alone at lunch.

That's servant leadership.

BEGIN AND END WITH GRATITUDE

Gratitude and service are connected.

Back in the chapter called "Telos" I explained how the Examen calls us to gratitude for each day's highs *and* lows—because both are part of the human experience and our pilgrim journey of growth as we make our path. And in "Machine Maintenance," I shared some thoughts about how gratitude can help us handle negative emotions. The Jesuits have taught me, right from the time I started high school, that it's good to begin and end everything we do with gratitude.

A kid once asked me why we pray before races. "I don't think God really cares who wins this race," he said, smirking. "Don't you think it's a little obnoxious to pray for victory?"

I had to laugh. "You're right. I don't think God really cares who wins this race. But I do think God cares deeply about the people in it. So let's pray with and for each other. And let's be grateful for the experience, win or lose."

Try to begin and end everything with gratitude—whether it's a championship race, just another day in math class, or eating dinner someone made for you. It'll help you be more appreciative of the people in your life. It'll help you take things less for granted. And it will help make you a man of service. Because service and gratitude are interconnected. One tends to lead to the other, in a continuous cycle of the good.

What Is Service?

Service is a broad term. It could mean anything from picking up trash to mowing an elderly neighbor's lawn to enlisting in the military. The earlier chapter on discerning a telos—a long-term vision for your life—suggested that living for some higher purpose helps us make our path toward virtue. It stands to reason, then, that service to others, including to society as a whole, is a crucial part of a telos oriented toward a higher purpose.

Developing an "ethic of service" means making generosity to others a default setting. Hopefully, we begin developing a willingness to be of service to others at a young age, because we are what we repeatedly do.

First of all, you have to take care of yourself if you want to help others—remember the story of the Two Foundations. You can't be much good to others if you're falling apart.

But assuming you are taking good care of yourself, you can then make a habit of serving others—that is, giving more than you take, like those seniors did. It eventually gets hardwired. You develop an ethic of service. It becomes a virtue.

We all need help developing the habit of service.

Service Learning

Sometimes, it takes some kind of organized program to kick-start that process. "Service learning" creates encounters between and among people, where we can learn to recognize and appreciate each other's humanity more deeply. Programs like these take you out of your comfort zone and set the stage for these encounters. They challenge you to work together toward a common "greater good." Often, these are required by schools or civic organizations. But is there really anything noble or generous about service if it's required?

Fair point, but there are all kinds of experiences you might never have if they weren't required of you. The whole point of a liberal arts education is to develop your ability to think by engaging you in a wide range of subjects, from the sciences to the arts and humanities. If you want a high school diploma or a college degree, you're going to need to work your way through subjects that might not be your thing.

The idea is that you can't know what "your thing" is unless you try lots of things.

Well, you can't develop a very meaningful "worldview" without viewing the world, either. Service learning is aimed at the gradual transformation of the learner. In that way, I suppose service learning isn't all that different from other education.

Except, it usually is.

In my experience, kids engage service work—and not just the work, but the *spirit* of the work—wholeheartedly. Sure, there is a camaraderie that emerges, and perhaps a sort of endorphin-fueled cheerfulness that comes from the satisfaction of being helpful to someone. But it's more than that. Often, guys who are normally sullen and withdrawn come out of their shells, embracing the sometimes tedious, repetitive work.

Of course, the work itself isn't the point—it's the relationships that emerge and the personal transformations that ensue.

I've taken a lot of guys on service trips, both closer to home and in far-off countries. Unmotivated kids discover a newfound energy and zest for life that doesn't fade when they come home. Guys who had small-minded, myopic attitudes about various issues find their perspectives radically shifted. I've seen insecure guys who had been living in fear of their own self-perceived inadequacies or failures rapidly develop a newfound sense of self-worth. Powerful connections happen.

While it might be common sense that doing something nice for someone else usually feels good, there's also plenty of research to suggest that engaging in service is good for us, including when it comes to mental health and wellbeing. Consider a 2023 study published in the *Journal of the American Medical Association*, which found that volunteering through some kind of organized group like a school or church is associated with better overall health and wellness for children and adolescents.[1] Likewise, a 2016 study from the University of Zurich in Switzerland using functional magnetic resonance imaging suggests a meaningful connection between generosity and mood-boosting effects at the neural level.[2]

SERVICE FAR AND NEAR

If you have the opportunity to participate in this type of immersive service program through a reputable, responsible agency, I encourage you to consider it. Even better if it involves some degree of travel, only because distance from what's familiar usually magnifies the impact.

The travel alone can constitute a transformative pilgrimage. Taking a challenging journey with a group of companions is a powerful and encouraging experience.

Your worldview will be more informed, because you'll be viewing the world beyond the familiar. You might learn another language, appreciate another cultural tradition, gain knowledge of a religious tradition, or develop a clearer understanding of global economics, wealth, and poverty.

Or maybe all of these things.

If it fits into your life at some point—and don't be so sure it can't—consider the possibility of engaging in some kind of extended service program. Some of the better-known of these (Peace Corps, AmeriCorps, the Jesuit Volunteer Corps, etc.) require a substantial commitment of time and involve a competitive application process. But there are many programs of differing types and durations offered through schools, universities, private secular foundations, and religious organizations. If you're in your late teens and twenties, do it now! Now is the time, before you might become settled more firmly into commitments like career, marriage, or fatherhood that will limit your flexibility.

Of course, opportunities like this aren't restricted to students or those just out of school. I can give you a very specific example. My longtime friend and colleague Adam Baber and I started a company called the Camino Institute in 2018. After having run international service programs for students together for many years, we realized that there was a desire on the part of adults to engage this type of experience. We had developed a lasting relationship with the community of El Faro in the central Dominican Republic—the village I told you about earlier, where we built the bridge. We returned there many times over the years, working with a particular foreman I've now known for almost twenty-five years.

We had some discussions with the community, raised some startup capital, and bought a couple acres of land there. We built a rustic hilltop retreat center overlooking the beautiful landscape where our clients come for weeklong service immersions. Our business model connects our groups with local workers to take on a small-scale construction project in the surrounding villages, usually benefiting either a family or the whole community. The clients we've worked with range from parents and their teenagers to grandparents in their sixties.

We do not have a savior complex; moreover, the community does not regard us in this way. We've built genuine, long-term, personal relationships. That's what good service organizations do. It is all about building relationships.

But you don't have to buy a plane ticket or devote a whole week to do a service program. There are plenty of ways to help charitable organizations wherever you are by volunteering. Local organizations have local knowledge, and that can maximize the reach of the good work you do. Whether it's lending a few hours of manual labor or helping a young child learn to read, service to others will carry a dual benefit: you'll help someone else while helping yourself.

EVERYDAY SERVANT LEADERSHIP

Organized service programs are important, but they are only part of the picture. Sometimes they encourage us to "measure the good" by racking up "service hours" or counting homes built or tabulating economic impact.

There's nothing intrinsically bad about that, but over time, it can skew our thinking about service—it can shape our understanding of it as something packaged and "taken care of" by checking these boxes. Certainly, that's not conducive to developing a "service ethic." It's sort of like, "Well, I already took care of my service obligation because I did *x*, so I guess I'm off the hook now."

If there's an opportunity to be of service in your everyday life—say, by stepping up at work or at home in a way that involves a little extra generosity on your part—you could see how you might pass it up if you're feeling smug about having just put in a ton of time and effort in an organized service program.

This would be ironic indeed.

What's the solution?

It's about balance, like almost everything else. We should invest ourselves in some organized service *and* do the small stuff of everyday life. Meeting our daily responsibilities is the first act of service—putting everyday effort into our homework, our jobs, our chores, our friendships, our marriages, our families, and our communities.

Finally, self-awareness, common decency, and good manners are basic forms of service. Things as simple as saying please and thank you are grounded in respect—and that's a bedrock of service. There is an old maxim that you can tell a lot about a person by the way they treat service employees like waiters, drivers, or cashiers. It isn't *just* about being polite, because politeness can be an act. Rather, I think it's about having the politeness that emerges from having *genuine* respect for people as your fellow human beings. A foundation of any service ethic, after all, is respect for people.

THE SERVICE OF MENTORSHIP

A great form of servant leadership that you can take on is mentorship. Whether it's through a community organization or just an informal relationship, maybe you can use your knowledge, experience, and wisdom to help out a younger person.

Could you serve as an assistant coach on a little league team?

Could you tutor neighborhood kids through a community center?

Could you just make an effort to look out for a younger person who seems to be struggling to fit in?

Taking on a mentoring role can be a rewarding and generous form of servant leadership—but it's also a serious responsibility. You have to bear in mind the limits of your knowledge and experience and not to try to be everything to someone.

For example, if you're helping out as an assistant coach and a kid could benefit from the wisdom and knowledge of a more experienced coach, you'll want to help them connect to that other source—not let pride at being a mentor get in the way.

Or, if a kid needs guidance with a serious issue, they might confide in you. There's a temptation to try to handle it on your own, but if it's over your head (or you're not sure if it is), the responsible thing to do is to find the right person who's qualified to help.

———

Back in 2004, sixteen years before Adam and I founded the Camino Institute, I spent a month in a small village in the Dominican Republic just a mile or so from the border with Haiti. This was a school-based service-learning program at Georgetown Prep, and I was there as a young faculty leader with two colleagues and a small group of guys between their junior and senior year.

One of those boys was radically transformed by his experience. It amounted to a pilgrimage of the body, mind, heart, and soul. This set in motion several years of deepening spirituality and service throughout college and beyond.

Eventually, he committed his life to the service of others with a religious vocation. We stayed in touch. Years after he'd made that trip with me, he sent a note expressing his gratitude. Within that note was a quote from Saint Mother Teresa of Calcutta: "I can do what you cannot, and you can do what I cannot. Together, we can do something beautiful for God." This was a touching tribute and an expression of gratitude I will never forget. Of course, the lifelong commitment to service that this young man made is the most rewarding thing of all.

Charity begets charity; service begets service.

The more you work at making service to others your default setting, the more it will become integrated into your everyday life. Having that kind of ethic boosts your self-awareness. It boosts your attention to others. It makes you a better companion, and it fosters generosity. Those are all good qualities to embrace as you make your path.

Chapter Thirteen

Wired Up

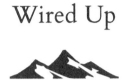

Remember D.J., my older brother's friend who traveled with us to Nepal? You know, the guy I called "human duct tape," who I said can fix just about anything and never seems to run out of patience and optimism?

I learned a lot from D.J. on that trip. Most of it was related to living in the present moment, which is something I wasn't very good at back then. The most memorable lesson was when D.J. introduced me to something he calls "The Stü." This is pronounced just like "stew," but The Stü is not edible. It's not even a thing at all, really. It's a state of being. And it's only spelled like that because D.J. says that makes it more exotic and mysterious.

Ridiculous, I know. But he insists.

The Stü is a state you enter when you intentionally do nothing. But can you intentionally do nothing? If it's intentional, then doesn't that mean you're doing something?

Good questions. The Stü is very mysterious.

During his many travels in developing countries, especially in remote areas, D.J. found himself doing a lot of waiting. At first, it was aggravating, and it collided with his can-do American mindset. But he learned that if you give yourself enough time in a culture accustomed to living a slower pace of life, you'll find yourself slowing down.

He found that by sitting quietly, and more or less motionless, he could enter a sort of meditative detachment from worry and concern.

It isn't *just* detachment, though. Because in The Stü you are also deeply aware of yourself and the world around you. All the different ingredients of life simmer, settle, and blend. After a while, all things become part of one another.

You know, like, in a stew.

I first learned to enter The Stü in that the Himalayan wilderness twenty-five years ago, sipping tea with Tom and D.J., overlooking the vast expanse of the rugged mountain landscape before us.

But once you discover The Stü, it's always with you, waiting to reconnect. I've entered The Stü in rugged, remote places, like the primeval Adirondack forest, the windswept plains of North Dakota, the vast desert plateaus of Arizona, and the glacial mountain passes of Patagonian Chile. Just as readily, though, I can find The Stü amid the bustling cacophony of a street market in the Dominican Republic or the frenetic hustle of an international airport terminal.

Perhaps most importantly, though, The Stü waits for you in everyday life. During the crazy, stressful, sleep-deprived years when my wife and I had three kids in diapers, I needed The Stü right there at home. Sometimes I find The Stü for just a few minutes, sipping coffee and watching the snow fall outside my window.

THE LOST ART OF BOREDOM

The Stü is the absence of action. It's peaceful boredom. Not tedious boredom, the kind that leaves you tapping your foot, feeling trapped in your own skin. It's a relaxing, energizing, peaceful state of having nothing in particular to do and being perfectly okay with that.

We need that sometimes.

That kind of boredom actually stirs the imagination.

Boredom teaches us that it's okay to spend time *not* achieving something.

That old kind of boredom lets your imagination run. It's the gray space in which we come up with new ideas. It's when we work through things in our head. It's the place for daydreaming. Without it, where do we daydream? Where do we exercise the imagination? And, moreover, without that kind of clear mental space at night, absent diversion and stimulation, how can we expect to fall asleep?

But now, it's almost impossible to get bored. At least not in the old way, when life involved less technology. That "old" kind of boredom came when there was nothing to do, or look at, or watch, or read. Now, when we're bored, it's often *despite* the limitless stimulation and choice of our digital technology.

Whether it's through games, media, other entertaining diversions, or the constant opportunity for productivity, one thing is clear: when we are wired up, the "old kind of boredom," the detachment, The Stü that we enter when we *lack* outside stimulation or diversion, is almost impossible.

DIGITAL TECHNOLOGY: A BLESSING AND A CURSE

I have a love-hate relationship with technology, and I'm guessing maybe you do, too.

I'm in my mid-forties, and I wasn't raised in an online world. That's where you and I—assuming you're in your teens, twenties, or maybe even early thirties—have the most radically different generational difference. Sure, I have warm memories of many hours spent playing video games, whether on our old school game console or the now-archaic desktop computer that ran on floppy disks. But it just wasn't that big a deal.

I'm not anti-technology. Digital tools fuel my creative pursuits, writing, publishing, and business growth. I make most of my income through remote editorial work that depends completely on such technologies.

But whether we're talking about my generation or yours, we know that for all its amazing features, digital technology is also a curse. In my experience, it's because of two traps: process addiction and obsession with productivity.

TRAP 1: PROCESS ADDICTION

There are two main categories of addiction: substance and process addiction. Substance addiction is what happens when we're compelled to use a substance of some kind, like a drug, and we don't have control of how we handle that compulsion. Process addiction, on the other hand, is when we're compelled to *do* something, like gamble or check our social media feed, and can't seem to control that drive.

Substance and process addiction aren't the same thing, of course, but they both function in similar ways—and they both involve dopamine. This is the chemical in the brain that drives us to do rewarding things—and ensures that both anticipating and doing those things is pleasurable. This goes back to biology and survival.

Think about food for a minute. The reason our biology has developed to enjoy satisfying flavors when we eat food is to encourage us to eat food—because we'll live longer if we do. The same goes for other things that help our survival odds: warmth feels good, quenching thirst feels good, being in the protective circle of family and friends feels good, and even getting the attention of a text message feels good.

Just as importantly, the *anticipation* of these things feels good—there's a preliminary "buzz," if you will, that comes in just knowing that the "high" is on the way. That's basically how dopamine works—by enticing and rewarding behaviors that, in their most essential raw form, our brains have determined are good for survival.

If you doubt this, try a little experiment. Take out your phone.

Check for notifications—but *don't* click on them.

Don't.

Click.

On.

Them.

Feel that tension right now? That's the tension of your dopamine-driven anticipatory excitement pulling against your self-control. (Okay, go ahead and check your notifications so you can get back here and focus.)

That felt good, didn't it?

Now put your phone down, and let's continue.

Dopamine is at the heart of habits because it connects directly with what scientists have come to understand about neuroplasticity—the fact that our brains rewire themselves based on conditions and repeated behaviors.

This is especially important to know when you're young, because the younger you are, the more plastic your brain is. It's busily wiring up patterns of anticipation and reward that tie in directly with our habits and behaviors. Put as simply as possible, the brain gets better at doing what it repeatedly does—especially where survival mechanisms are involved.

What does all this have to do with process addiction? Well, dopamine is potent stuff, and it can work against us sometimes as it drives us to pursue pleasurable things.

Those same survival mechanisms tied in with dopamine encourage the brain to seek novelty. This makes sense. Too much of one thing isn't good for survival of the species, whether it's too much of the same genetic mating pool or too much of a single food.

So, it stands to reason that the anticipatory and pleasure-reward circuitry of the brain would *prefer* novelty, variety, and change. If we haven't had a chocolate bar in a while, a chocolate bar is very appealing. If we have a chocolate bar handed to us every day for a week, it's going to be *decreasingly* appealing; however, if on day eight, we are suddenly handed a bag of something different, like gummy bears, those gummy bears are going to skyrocket in terms of their appeal.

We get turned on, neurologically speaking, by novelty—and the more novelty and variety we are presented with, the more our brains take advantage of that by rewarding it.

Think of how much novelty our digital devices afford us.

A *lot*.

Streaming platforms, video games, and nearly endless variety. There is limitless diversion at our fingertips. Whether it's through massively multiplayer online gaming, lighthearted apps on our phones, or realistic digital simulations, we have the opportunity to immerse ourselves in a hyperstimulating, ever-changing dynamic world of entertainment. (Porn, of course, is one element of that world—see the next chapter.)

Social media platforms create a different form of entertainment and diversion. While they aren't specifically designed as games, there is a gamified element to them: they draw us in to an immersive ecosystem of stimulating information, stories, and experiences.

A dependency on variety means that there is an endless and relentless need for it, and it's a self-perpetuating cycle. The more variety is presented, the more variety is desired, and the less desire there is for "the same old thing."

Over time, this cycle of training the brain to anticipate and experience novel stimuli, afforded through the limitless stream of unlimited digital content, can get us totally hooked on our screens. That's a serious trap, and if you have a smartphone, you probably already know about it.

The good news is that neuroplasticity works in all directions. If you want to change a habit, you can do it. Your brain gets better at what you repeatedly do. Of course, you might need to set some rules to get the change started, but you already know that.

Of course, a few hacks here and there might be helpful, too. One effective strategy to reduce habitual or compulsive smartphone use is to change your smartphone's display to black and white. This makes it considerably less interesting to look at. I realize it sounds a little silly, since you can always just switch it back to full color. Someone suggested this to me, and I was skeptical of it too. But I tried it, and I was surprised just how effective it turned out to be. I ran a little experiment and did this for three days. Then I looked at my screen time for those days compared to my average. I was surprised by how much lower it was. Maybe give it a try, at least during school or work hours when you're trying to be productive.

Trap 2: Prioritizing Productivity

The other trap is the "productivity trap."

It's one thing to avoid excess of something that society tends to frown upon, such as a more visibly harmful substance or behavior, like problem gambling. There are plenty of messages discouraging this. It's another thing entirely to avoid excess of something that is inherently praiseworthy, like getting stuff done.

We can become addicted to work. To producing content, doing our jobs, checking boxes, and generating value. These are all things that aren't bad on their own merits, but like anything else in excess, they can become toxic. With collaboration and productivity apps increasingly cloud-based and omnipresent, the school day or workday no longer has a clear end. Just as social media and news apps provide the dilemma of the endless feed, the hyperconnected workplace follows us everywhere we let it.

When there isn't a clear divide between our classrooms, lecture halls, workplaces, or offices and our bedrooms, we shouldn't be surprised that we're treading on potentially dangerous ground when it comes to keeping things balanced.

This is a particularly nasty little problem, this productivity trap, because productivity is broadly considered a virtue in our culture. I'm not suggesting that it isn't—but I am inviting you to consider this in light of the previous discussion of balance and excess. What does excess productivity look like? Well, for one thing, it's sure to interfere with relationships, as getting stuff done consistently takes precedence over relationship-building.

If you aren't sure what this would look like, just envision a couple at a restaurant, each distracted by a phone. If it's happening at the dinner table, it's happening everywhere else, too. The tough part is that it all seems justifiable. That one text or email is important, sure. It's when we zoom out and look at patterns of excess that it becomes a problem.

NAVIGATING SOCIAL MEDIA: LESS IS MORE

When I think back to my boyhood in the 1980s and 1990s, very few of my memories involve screens. Whenever they did, the screens were most often at the center of a *communal* experience: playing video games with my brothers or friends, or watching a movie together. There was no internet; we had no phones. If you were to travel back in time to 1996, find my friends and me hanging out after school, and try to explain today's social media landscape to us at age sixteen, we would have looked at you like you were insane. We would have told you that sounds like the most unbelievable waste of time we could imagine.

Furthermore, we would have told you that if anyone tried using a device that could take pictures or video of our social lives and then share it, more or less permanently, for *the entire world to see*, we would have made sure to (1) destroy that device very quickly and (2) stay far away from any such lunatic who would think for two seconds that this would *ever* be a good idea.

And then we would have gone back to whatever it was we were doing together. That might have been as mundane as hanging out and renting a VHS movie, and wishing we weren't losers watching movies on a Friday night, or it might have been as exciting as cruising around at night, and going to the mall, or going to a stupid party and then wishing we hadn't. But the point is, we were always *together*. Not "together" online, but actually together. We were a friend group, but we didn't call it a friend group. None of us had a phone, but we were *tight*, man.

Enough has been written about social media that it would take anyone a lifetime to read even a portion of it. Unless you've been living under a rock, you no doubt have been part of conversations about its influence on contemporary society—and there's a good chance it's already a part of your life. I'm a strong proponent of the philosophy that young kids and social media are a bad combination. (Entire books have been written about that by some pretty smart people.) But if you're an older teenager or young adult, it's almost inevitable that you'll make use of it.

Like so many other things, the key to healthy relationship with social media is moderation. Perhaps you want to keep your life free of social media, which is both admirable and difficult. There's a part of me that would like to endorse that as the best approach, and embrace the now-ubiquitous phrase associated with drug abuse education: "Just say no." The problem with that approach is that in the twenty-first century, it just might not be practical. You may find that you are missing out on opportunities, both social and professional, depending on your field. I do think it's possible to use social media in an intelligent, productive way.

My suggestion is that you limit the number of accounts you maintain. First of all, each one is another channel for distraction and addiction. Second, each one presents another digital minefield with the real potential to explode in a reputational catastrophe—even if you're careful. Some of the apps are more or less professional; others are clearly more of a playground.

I find that social media has been useful for business purposes. Insofar as it has helped me share my writing, build my readership, and advertise my editorial services, it's been a powerful and effective tool. It's also been very good for spreading the word about the Camino Institute—sharing photos and videos, directing interested people to our website. But I've found it less appealing for personal use. I used to use it to make more personal, day-to-day, casual posts. Not anymore. I find that line in the sand has been helpful, and it's reduced the amount of time I waste scrolling through various feeds. Maybe that approach might work for you.

Another suggestion is to avoid commenting on others' posts, except to offer occasional positive feedback and affirmation. If you find yourself driven to submit something critical, controversial, or antagonistic, think twice. The momentary satisfaction you might feel from firing off a zinger in response to a post is not going to last amid the miserable experience of social media mob-shaming. It can happen very fast and get very ugly. No doubt you've already seen it happen. As I've said to students many times, a good rule of thumb to follow before you post anything online, on any platform:

1. Imagine three people. One you love deeply, one who is in a position of official authority over you, and one whose opinion of you has bearing on your reputation. For example: your mom, your principal, and your boss.

2. Imagine all three of them seeing this post and knowing it was yours.

3. If you hesitate at all because of one, two, or all three of them—even just a little bit—then *don't post it.* Either shut down the app and go do something else or edit/revise the post until you'd be okay with *all three of them* seeing it.

Anyone who uses social media—and I mean anyone, whether fifteen or fifty—absolutely must understand something first. That is that once you post something online, it's *published.* It's public. It's out there, and deleted or not, screenshots are forever. (That's why I so strongly believe that young kids shouldn't use it at all. The stakes are just too high.) That means you need to navigate the social media landscape the same way you'd drive on a busy freeway. Enjoy the ride, but always practice defensive driving. Slow down. Don't tailgate. Don't provoke other drivers. And never forget how quickly things can go wrong if you're not careful.

Disconnect to Reconnect

If you'll think back on the chapter about "Getting to Virtue," you'll recall that we considered how we first need rules to build good habits, which might, eventually, become habituated moral behaviors—which is how we defined virtues. That first part, about the rules, is crucial. Put another way—and I think this is really important when it comes to gaining control over addictive technology—we have to start with *the imposition of rules*.

A half-hearted effort to build positive habits (or break negative ones) just won't work. I can't "kind of" stop eating late-night snacks. I can't "kind of" commit to doing twenty minutes of exercise each day. If I "kind of" commit to something, I'll "kind of" habituate it. This is where I think we have to have the humility to recognize our own limits when it comes to self-discipline, and the very important role that firm rules have in that regard.

If you are finding an imbalance when it comes to being "wired up," such that you're feeling an excess of stimulation, then you have to establish some rules. Take an honest look at how much of your life is dominated by technology, ask yourself if you're happy with the answer, and if you're not, then make some rules.

Maybe even just one rule.

Then figure out how to hold yourself accountable to the rule(s). This probably involves telling someone about your rule(s) and asking that person to give you a gentle kick in the butt when you break them. Your rules will probably have to change. That's fine. Just don't stop thinking of them as rules, because as soon as you do that, they won't work.

One rule I have is that I don't look at my phone in the morning until I've first taken at least a few minutes to make a cup of coffee and drink it. Unless the weather really doesn't allow it, I do so outside, looking at the tree in front of my house and listening to the birds.

It works because it's simple and it isn't demanding that much. The days when I follow that rule are, without exception, better than ones when I don't. Because sometimes I break the rule and look at my phone first thing. Because I'm human. It happens. At least when it does, though, I know I've broken my rule, and I feel that. I think of the birds I didn't listen to, and I feel a little pang of regret. I mean, I like those birds.

WILDERNESS THERAPY

If you're not too keen on all this business about making rules, let me offer another way to tackle the "always connected" problem: Just get outside. Edward Abbey, in his famous work *Desert Solitaire*, may have said it best:

> *So get out there and hunt and fish and mess around with your friends, ramble out yonder and explore the forests, climb the mountains, bag the peaks, run the rivers, breathe deep of that yet sweet and lucid air, sit quietly for a while and contemplate the precious stillness, the lovely, mysterious, and awesome space.*[1]

Spend time in the wilderness and, if possible, extend this to places you have to reach on foot. If outdoor stuff like hiking, camping, and the like is "not your thing," I get that. But I'd also encourage you to reconsider giving it a try, because like anything else that you've determined is "not your thing," maybe it actually could be if you were open to the possibility.

On a shoestring budget, I took a five-week, 11,500-mile summer road trip all around the United States with my friend Kary when we were both in our early twenties. I did the same thing, although over a little less distance, and just for two weeks, with my friend Scott in my late twenties. Both were extraordinary journeys, and they include some of my most cherished memories from that time of my life. Our National Parks here in the United States do not disappoint. Get out there and see them when and if you can.

Traveling in this way is money well spent—far more so than tourist packages and pricey vacations. For the same investment you might spend on a booze-fueled week at an overcrowded beach club or gambling excursion to Las Vegas, you can rent a car for a few weeks and set out on a true odyssey with a few good friends seeing the country up close and exploring some of the most beautiful wilderness on earth.

If you decide to make this kind of pilgrimage, do enough planning as to make good use of your time, but don't over-plan. Get yourself a paper road atlas and use that instead of GPS unless you need it. Oh. And your phones? Here's a super-crucial thing. Either turn them off completely unless needed for emergencies or take measures to reduce the distractions. That might mean deleting your social media apps—or at the very least, turning off notifications. Sure, it's great to have a camera, a phone, a map, and a flashlight when you're traveling. And the great thing is, with a few quick settings, you can limit your phone to those amazing tools without all the other distractions.

—⁓—

The retreats we run at our school are popular. These overnight trips invite guys to get real about where they've been, where they are, and where they want to go. They're powerful bonding experiences—the sort of "rite of passage" I mentioned earlier.

One of the rules we have is no electronic devices. At first, it's an adjustment, and some of them grumble as they hand over their phones. But by the end, everyone is grateful that we do it. When they're sitting around a campfire, deep in conversation, opening up about stuff buried deep in their hearts, they realize the freedom that comes with unplugging.

Several years back, I was skipping stones with a group of juniors on the lake in front of the retreat house. It was the second night of an October retreat, and the sky was on fire with a beautiful sunset. One of guys turned to me and said, "It's pretty ironic. You took away all our devices, but this is the most connected we've ever been."

I smiled, because I knew he'd found The Stü.

Chapter Fourteen

Hormones and Habits

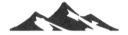

WHEN I WAS IN MY TWENTIES, I was chaperoning our high school ski club. I always enjoyed this role, because I got to ski, have dinner with fellow teachers, and spend some time in a casual setting with students, both on the chartered bus trip and on the slopes. On the hour-long ride home, I would get a chance to chat with kids about all sorts of stuff—at least when they weren't glued to their phones. Mostly we'd talk about school, sports, or their future plans. Sometimes they'd ask me about places I'd traveled to or other life experiences. Occasionally, the conversations would go a little deeper. One time, a group of students that I also happened to coach on the rowing team were huddled in what appeared to be an intense conversation a few rows back. I heard, "Ask him! Go ahead! Don't worry. He's cool; you can ask him." A reluctant emissary shuffled forward and asked if I could handle a weird question. I shrugged and told him, "I guess."

He motioned for me to follow and headed back to his seat. Unsure what I was in for, and bracing for anything, I made my way back to where they were seated. I stood in the aisle and leaned in as the boldest of the group, in a hushed voice, asked, "Coach, um, is it okay if a guy checks out porn and, you know, does what guys do? Like, every day?"

Well, I may have braced for anything, but I was not in any way prepared for this question—so I did what young teachers often do when something throws them for a loop. I panicked. I rolled my eyes and said something like, "Uh, why don't you ask your dad that one?" before going back to my row in the bus. I could hear them muttering their disappointment. The messenger, slumping back into his seat, chirped at the others, "I told you! Now it's weird." After a minute of thinking it over, I realized that this was what we in the education business refer to as a "teachable moment," and that I had squandered it by being dismissive. It was a genuine question, and my students trusted me enough as a coach, teacher, and mentor to ask it.

I focused my thoughts, took a deep breath, and walked back there again. They abruptly stopped talking and looked out the window, embarrassed. "Okay. You guys really want my answer?" I asked. They did. They weren't kidding around. They'd actually posed two separate questions. One was about "checking out porn" and the other was about "doing what guys do" with porn. These two activities are obviously related, but they're not the same thing.

So, I said what I think. First, that masturbation (yeah, they cringed at the word; but hey, they asked) is just part of growing up, and some people make a bigger deal out of it than they should. I told them it was a response to hormones, and that testosterone is potent stuff. I acknowledged it's something almost all guys do when they're teenagers. Of course, they already knew that.

That said, I also wanted to say something about the Church's teaching on the matter. I thought that was important, as a teacher at their Catholic school. I told them that while I don't think it's good to make a big deal about it, it's likewise a mistake to think it doesn't matter at all. I told them I think the problem is that it makes sexuality all about pleasure, without any commitment to a relationship, any sacrifice, or any self-discipline. People end up getting objectified. After all, the images and scenarios that tend to accompany this activity—whether conjured up in the sexual imagination or viewed in pornography—are not flattering ones. They make people a means to an end.

Oh, and there's also a catch that I think most guys understand: it's habit-forming.

I told them I understand that self-control in this area is pretty tough when your hormones are on overdrive as a teenager. I suggested that, like so many other things in life, you just have to do your best and try to stick to the high road as you navigate your way through this part of growing up. I told them I think they'd find that those impulses might actually get a little *more* challenging to manage as the testosterone keeps rising for the next few years—but that eventually, things would calm down in that department.

But then there was their other question. The one about whether it was okay to watch porn. I told them I think that's a different proposition, and that no, I don't think it's okay. I told them I think there's a significant difference between doing something guys have been doing forever—something that's just part of growing up—and venturing into the realm of online porn. Internet porn totally changes the game, because it takes things too far and it's potentially addictive. I left it at that, because I didn't really have anything else to say and because the bus trip was almost over anyway. They seemed to be taking what I said seriously, and they thanked me. As I drove home, I got to thinking just how tricky it must be to be a teenager in the age of the internet, and I hoped my attempt to answer their questions was helpful.

This topic used to be relegated to private talks about the birds and the bees, or perhaps the hushed confines of the confessional. And maybe that was enough said about it before the internet totally transformed the landscape of adolescence, including infusing it with exposure to porn. But now, this issue has become much more prominent in the public discourse, and for good reason. Researchers, social scientists, psychologists, addiction counselors, and medical professionals are chiming in on the matter. Concern about the impact of porn on teens and adults alike has extended beyond the private confines of the confessional to the arena of addiction science, psychosexual development, marriage, and even public health. I think these concerns are important for guys to understand.

RECOGNIZING THE PROBLEM OF PORN

Where does the word "pornography" come from? The ending "-graphy" refers to mapping. So, "geography" means "mapping the earth" and photography means "mapping the light," specifically different wavelengths of light. *Pornos* is Greek for prostitute—thus pornography is a very old word that means "mapping the prostitute." A prostitute is one paid and used by another in a sexual context. There's a transactional relationship involved. A deep question for any guy to consider, if and when he uses pornography, is to ask: who is using whom, exactly, and what's the cost?

It's worth mentioning that the conversation on the ski bus took place not long after the first smartphones came out. Only some of them had the devices at that point, which meant that only some of them had the internet with them at all times, on a private little screen of their own. Within the next couple of years, I would find myself working at a school full of guys carrying smartphones, their lives increasingly enmeshed in the digital landscape. As time went on, I had more frequent conversations, with both students and colleagues, about the challenges presented by the constant presence of electronic devices and the digital world they connect us to.

Like any other school, we soon wrestled with digital distraction, social media, excessive gaming, and inappropriate online behaviors—all parts of being "wired up," which we discussed in the previous chapter. At a school full of teenage boys, we became increasingly aware of the reality that online porn was something we had a responsibility to address. When we broached the topic directly in a meeting of administrators and counselors focused on student life, I found myself thinking back to that conversation on the ski bus. At that point, I'd had no idea how familiar an issue this would become in the years ahead.

We consulted with some experts in male development. We examined some of the existing scientific research. We invited a group of mature student leaders to offer their perspectives and insights. It's worth noting that the students in those early conversations were adamant that this was, in fact, a real issue that guys their age were wrestling with. They were strongly in favor of our taking some kind of action to broach this topic and provide some guidance on it, as uncomfortable as it might be. They helped us build an anonymous survey, which we then refined with people trained in survey methodology. This gave us some baseline data to start with. Through a lot of hard work and no small bit of institutional courage, we got a program off the ground. It's been going strong for a number of years now. Faculty and peer mentors invite guys to understand this topic, talk about it openly and honestly, understand the moral and ethical implications, and learn strategies for navigating their journey of sexual development without getting hooked on internet porn.

At first, this was uncharted territory. But like other difficult topics, we've found that the more directly we address the problem of porn, the less tricky it is to have meaningful conversations about it. As the years have progressed, more and more schools have begun taking action to address this topic, and it has become increasingly evident that many teenage guys struggle with this. The reality is, however, that habitual porn use is not confined to the teenage demographic. Plenty of young—and not so young—men are hooked, too.

THE TENSION BETWEEN BIOLOGY AND CULTURE

Any guy who has lived through adolescence knows that there are few forces on the planet as persistent as sex drive. Without it, we wouldn't last too long. It's an evolutionary mechanism essential to the survival of the species. Accordingly, high sex drive correlates with peak physical development in the late teen and young adult years. Biologically, that's when we're at our fittest—so it makes sense, biologically, to reproduce.

Yet biology changes at a glacially slow pace compared to culture. Our religions and cultures encourage reproduction in the responsible context of marriage, but biological brains haven't caught up. They still urge us to get busy as teenagers. There's the adolescent conundrum: just as the brain and body kick into hormonal overdrive to ensure continuity of the species, our cultural and religious norms discourage sex—again, for many good reasons.

Talk about tension, man. You don't need advanced knowledge of psychosexual development to know how most young guys handle it. While statistical data on such a taboo topic is limited, there is enough to substantiate what everyone knows anyway. If you really feel the need for some scientific validation, you can look at research from more than a dozen years ago (2011) in the *Journal of the American Medical Association*, which noted that 80 percent of seventeen-year-old males involved in the study reported having masturbated.[1] (In other news, the sun is hot.) Moreover, 2011 was a technological lifetime ago, before almost every teenager in the world was carrying a smartphone that gave them practically unlimited access to porn. While formalized research like this seeks to "prove" it, the fact that young guys do this a lot is not exactly a secret. Or, if it is, it's probably the worst-kept secret ever.

RELIGIOUS TEACHINGS AND SELF-CONTROL

While the specifics vary, the wisdom expressed in many religious teachings is, basically, that masturbation is wrong because it separates sex from love. It makes your sexual response all about yourself while you objectify others in your imagination. At the same time, it reduces your appreciation for the sanctity of your sexuality—along with objectifying others, it objectifies yourself. Now, you might not agree with this, but I think you can at least agree that habitual masturbation gradually changes the way a guy thinks about sex, his body, and other people's bodies—and not in a particularly respectful way.

Whatever you believe—even if you have no formal religious identity—you might appreciate the self-discipline that such religious admonitions call us to practice. You might consider trying to resist sexual urges—or at least moderate how much you choose to respond to them—even if for no other reason than to practice self-control. After all, if you can maintain control over such a powerful drive in private, it proves you are capable of self-discipline in other areas of your life, too. That's a way to build integrity.

A high school senior talked to me about this a few years back. He explained that he was frustrated because despite being super disciplined in every other area of his life, this was the one area where he felt totally unable to control himself. Obviously, this guy was pretty confident—not every kid has the wherewithal to have that conversation, even with a trusted mentor. That should make it even more clear that this is something even the most put-together guys might struggle with.

Why did something so typical to his age bother him so much? The moral implications bothered him, sure, but he was mostly ticked that he couldn't be in control of something so simple. He was a leader and a go-getter; he was reliable, honest, and kind. He was a leader on the field and in the classroom. He endured grueling workouts to achieve an excellent physique. He'd made all kinds of disciplined sacrifices to earn the grades to gain admission to a top-tier college. He even had a beautiful girlfriend. So why couldn't he get control over this, he wondered? Why, when it came to this, did he feel like a kid unable to resist another piece of candy? We talked a little more, and it probably won't surprise you to hear that it had a lot to do with the porn he'd be watching since—get this—age eleven.

The following year, he stopped by school when he was home on spring break from college. He was happy. We talked about his major and his professors. I wasn't going to bring up the conversation we'd had a year earlier. After a little while, he turned to leave my office. But before he did, he lowered his voice and told me that hey, by the way, he was happy to say he'd gotten control over that part of his life. The key was quitting porn.

Too Much, Too Soon, Too Often

Prior to the internet going mainstream, porn was a lot harder for a kid to find. There were several "barriers to entry," not the least of which was the legal age requirement to purchase a magazine from the corner store or a VHS tape from some sketchy video outlet by the freeway. Typically, a kid's supply of porn consisted of one or two crumpled back issues of a glossy magazine tucked away somewhere in his room.

The internet changed everything because of three things: accessibility, quantity, and explicitness. Porn is easier to get, there's a limitless supply of it, and it's a lot more intense. As a result, porn has become an insidious thing in the life of today's smartphone-equipped boys and young men. A nonreligious, nonlegislative, nonprofit organization in the United States called Fight the New Drug[2] has conducted numerous studies and curated data from a broad body of research. A quick visit to its website will provide many statistics. For example, in a 2021 study of American teens aged fourteen to eighteen, 84 percent of males had viewed pornography compared to 57 percent of females.[3] In conjunction with speaking engagements and seminars I've offered at several independent boys' high schools over the past decade, I have conducted additional surveys similar to that original one I mentioned, each aiming to garner insights into young men's behaviors, attitudes, and feelings associated with online life. While these surveys are less scientifically robust than formal studies by professional researchers and involve sample sizes of several hundred rather than tens of thousands, they are still informative. Each round of these surveys has suggested that well over half of high-school-aged boys are regular consumers of online porn.

Another revealing insight in the surveys I've conducted is that most respondents report their first exposure to pornography occurred *before* they were in high school. A more formal 2017 study involving 914 Australians aged fifteen to twenty-nine suggested the median age when boys first viewed pornography was thirteen.[4]

So, what does this mean? For many a boy growing up today, it's this: Just at the age when he is *least* equipped to handle powerful temptations due to his still-developing prefrontal cortex, unlimited porn comes flooding into his digital life, free of charge. This is like putting a five-year-old kid in a room full of candy, alone, and closing the door. Of course he's going to gorge on candy. And as long as that unlocked room full of candy is there, what's to stop him from going back for more?

Some boys seek out porn as much to learn about sex as to satisfy their own urges, and there's something innocent about that. This may be even more of a factor among boys who are unsure about their sexuality, for whom mainstream sex education and messaging may well be lacking or noninclusive. But porn makes a lousy sex-ed teacher: whatever it's depicting is almost certainly going to be unrealistic and objectifying. And even if there's an innocent motivation for watching it, well, sex ed should not come with a side of process addiction.

Now, I have to pause here to say that technically, addiction has a particular definition and that only qualified experts can formally diagnose one. There has been some debate in the scientific community as to whether to formally classify the type and frequency of pornography use that seems like an addiction as, in fact, an addiction. But some researchers support this classification, including the authors of a 2015 study in Switzerland, which, according to its abstract, "leads to the conclusion that Internet pornography addiction fits into the addiction framework and shares similar basic mechanisms with substance addiction."[5] Either way, I am no such expert. So, when I use the term addiction here, I'm using it in a layman's capacity, not in a clinical sense—although I mean simply this: something that has become so habitual that it's really hard to stop doing. I think it's fair to say that someone can be in that situation without having a *formally* diagnosed addiction.

So, with that said: Imagine you had the nefarious task of designing the perfect potential addiction. How would you build it? First off, you'd want it to be intensely rewarding— it has to feel good. You'd also want it to tap into a reward/ pleasure center that's universal—you wouldn't want to limit it only to one category of people—maximum reach would be better. You'd want it to be more or less physically harmless, so there was no obvious reason to stop. You'd want it to be legal (at least for adults). You'd also want it to be free of any obvious visible side effects, so that it wouldn't call attention to itself. You'd want to be sure it was easy, without much of a learning curve—a complicated process is unlikely to be too addictive. You'd also want it to be widely accessible—in fact, you'd want it to be practically free. Get the picture?

Compounding the problem is the fact that almost nobody is talking to kids about this issue, unlike drugs, alcohol, or sex itself. So, it's actually like giving that little boy access to that candy-filled room and not even telling him too much sugar is bad for him. Online porn presents a reliable pleasure-reward cycle unlike anything else a boy or young man has ever known, and it doesn't ask for anything in return—at least it seems that way. But like I said before, there's a catch. The catch is that porn has all the ingredients to be the perfect habit builder, especially for young guys.

THE HYPERSEXUALIZED BRAIN

Earlier on, in the chapter on "The Integrated Man," we dug into the term "toxic masculinity." We looked at the problems with that term, but we considered how "hypersexuality" could throw off a guy's balance.

A reasonable person can connect a steady diet of porn to hypersexuality. This is a highly stimulating, readily available, habit-forming product that hypersexualizes men *and* women, but often portrays the sexual domination and objectification of women. This builds toxicity into male sexuality.

Many middle-school-aged boys are watching extremely explicit porn, presumably becoming accustomed and desensitized to it through habituated masturbation, theoretically building up an association between sexual response and depraved scenarios absent anything resembling respectful, loving relationships, and then joking crudely about it, both online and in locker rooms. This pattern intensifies as they become teenagers.

The resulting desensitization to all things sexual has dangerous implications. A long-term porn habit can skew sexual attitudes, making a guy careless and cavalier about sex. Perhaps even worse, aggressive sexual behaviors, like the ones depicted in hardcore porn, can be normalized. There are frightening implications around how common it has become (at least anecdotally) for teenagers to exchange "nudes," which has massive implications, both ethical and legal.

Since most of the population is heterosexual, who are those most likely to bear the consequences of this skewed, desensitized, hypersexuality on the part of boys and men? It's obvious: girls and women. Examples of this are all over the media, and you don't have to look far to see young men behaving badly in the sexual realm—usually to the detriment of girls and women.

Take the situation that played out some years ago among one well-known university's men's athletic team. Some of the male students created a "roster" comprising members of the women's team, rating individuals with regard to various sexual criteria, some of it described in obscene and graphic detail.

The statistics surrounding sexual assault and rape are even more horrifying. Obviously, watching porn doesn't make one a criminal or future rapist. But it is naïve to dismiss the correlation between a hypersexualized population of boys and young men and a rise in inappropriate, disrespectful, and criminal sexual behavior—often directed at girls and women. An adolescence or young adulthood full of porn isn't going to help any guy develop into a sexually mature man. There's a strong case to be made that it may complicate that journey.

HYPERSEXUALIZED BODY IMAGE

A steady porn habit hypersexualizes body image, too. Girls and women have been feeling this pressure for a long time. For years, everything from magazine covers to underwear ads to porn magazines has conveyed an "ideal" female form, and the struggle to meet these unrealistic expectations has wrought havoc on teen girls especially, creating body image anxiety that often plays out in eating disorders and unhealthy diets.

Lately, though, there are signs that boys and men are struggling more openly with body image issues. There is more pressure than ever to rock that six-pack. Protein shakes, creatine, and other muscle-building supplements are now standard fare among high school athletes. According to medical experts, one of the problems common among boys is "muscle dysmorphia," which is characterized by a desire to bulk up or achieve more muscular definition. Perhaps unsurprisingly, for boys and men it's about a desire to be bigger—more or less the opposite of what drives the eating disorders more typical among girls and women.

That group of students that worked with us in developing the program we teach at school explained that porn has contributed to this body image anxiety among guys. One of them put it like this (I'm paraphrasing): We all know guys have always been obsessed with how they, you know, "measure up." Now, starting in middle school, boys are comparing themselves to what they see on screen. And how many guys measure up to that?

Perhaps it's no wonder that many boys and younger men these days think it's weird to be naked in a locker room. The more our culture connects nakedness intrinsically to sex, the more the two become inextricably linked. The irony speaks for itself: Much of the same generation of young adults that has been exposed to more pornographic media than any in history—the same generation for which the exchange of "nudes" has become a distressingly "normal" practice—is weirdly uncomfortable being naked around other people of the same sex for a few minutes.

An Exploitative Industry

There are voices out there that claim porn is harmless, and that the only reason it has such a stigma is because outdated religious traditions foster so much guilt about it. That there wouldn't be any guilt if it weren't for archaic religious mores. They'll say this is simply a chicken or egg question—that the guilt comes from the *teaching*, not from the porn. But the answer isn't that simple. Porn does harm people. It exploits those involved in the industry that produces it, and it affects those who use it, too. The pornography industry fits the very definition of *exploitation*: the unfair and uncaring use of one party by another for purposes of profit or gain.

The exploitation is there on many levels: most obviously of those involved as actors and those who, through sex trafficking, find themselves unwitting participants in the production of porn. To be clear, some actors embrace their roles, and a small minority are no doubt well-paid. At best, they are voluntarily dehumanized and reduced to avatars for sexual objectification. The great majority are not well paid, though, and many are subjected to abusive treatment, both physical and emotional.

The reality is that porn makes people into products. And that includes both the user and the actors. Both become "commodities" in a bad business. Why is it a bad business? Because it's exploitative. It *uses* people in a way that reduces them to mechanisms for cheap gratification that comes from impulsive cravings. And it does so with no regard for the addictive nature of the medium. I think it looks kind of like this:

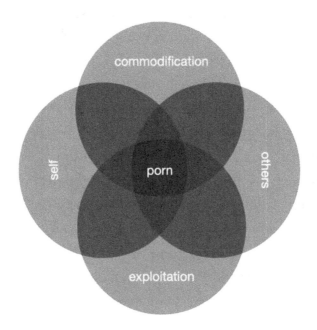

Bottom line? It is a multibillion-dollar industry fueled by sexual objectification. It commodifies people and exploits cravings. It seems to have all the ingredients to set the stage for addiction. And I can tell you, from quite a few conversations about it with guys over the years, it leads to a lot of self-loathing. All of that is to say that any man—especially one aiming for moral virtue— should steer clear of it.

Balance and Moderation

Okay. That's all well and good, but porn is tempting, and it's *right there*. How do you navigate this part of your journey?

First, acknowledge that your sexual attitudes and behaviors matter. This is a big part of who you are, and you shouldn't look at it as arbitrary or without consequence. Second, it comes down to discernment. Know what your genuine desires are and be able to differentiate them from impulsive cravings. Be honest with yourself about your drives and impulses, and don't immediately judge them as bad or good. Instead, consider how they make you feel. How do you handle them? Does this lead you to consolation or desolation?

Take an integrated look. This is clearly a "body" issue, but what does your mind, heart, and soul have to do with your drives and how you handle them?

I think most men would agree routine masturbation has been, and will remain, a typical behavior for teenage boys and young men, and that total abstinence from it is unlikely—at least up until a certain stage of life when the impulse is simply not so powerful. But *aiming* for self-control in this regard is a good idea. Take the sexual overstimulation of porn out of your life, and isn't it reasonable to assume sex—and, eventually we'd hope, the type of committed, loving relationship that should be intrinsic to it—will take on a greater value?

Of course, if you have any deeply ingrained habit, be patient with yourself. Change is hard. It takes time. Think of my dad's patient who lost a hundred pounds, starting with a single lap around his dining room table. Don't underestimate small improvements. If you watch porn seven days a week, try cutting down to six. That's a victory. Not a complete victory, no. You're still a guy who watches porn six days a week. But guess what? It's a victory because you'll have made a change that will encourage you. You'll have proved to yourself that *you're* in charge, not the porn. Give yourself some credit for that. Maybe the next week, you get it down to four days, and so on, and within a matter of weeks, you've put it behind you. There are two victories here: First, you've knocked porn out of your life. But second—and maybe more importantly—you've realized how capable you are of self-discipline and change.

I suppose all this comes down to a simple question for a guy trying to get a better handle on self-control when it comes to all of this: Navigating the journey of sexual maturity is hard enough already. Does porn really need to be a part of it?

—————

I was catching up over a beer with a guy I used to coach. He was in his early twenties, but he'd been a student when we first started offering our talks about the problems with porn. He asked if we still offered that program at school.

When I told him we did, he opened up and told me the story of how he'd been hooked on porn since middle school, but he'd never had the courage to talk to anyone about it. By midway through high school, he explained, he felt like a drug addict.

So, he'd sat in that classroom and listened, terrified of saying a word. He almost spoke up but couldn't muster the courage. It got worse in college. At one point, he discovered he couldn't even get aroused without porn. That's when he finally sought professional counseling. He met with a professional who *was* qualified to clinically classify his habit as a form of addiction. It took work, but he was happy to have turned things around in a matter of months.

There's a guy aiming for virtue, trying to make the "average tendency" of his path a little better. He had the humility to own up to something that was leading him astray and causing imbalance. He had the courage to ask for help. He had the discipline to change, little by little, until he was back on the path he wanted to travel.

Chapter Fifteen

Work, Money, and Freedom

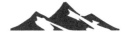

LIKE A LOT OF KIDS of my generation, my first job was delivering newspapers. It was simple, but it wasn't easy. I started at age nine, helping my older brother Peter unofficially, and then took over the route at eleven, when I was officially old enough. Most child employment is more strictly limited to older teenagers, but newspaper carriers are one of the exceptions.

Buffalo winters are tough, and the nasty weather lasts at least from mid-November through late March—and that's in a good year. For months, my weekend mornings and afterschool hours were spent slogging through snow or cold rain with a heavy satchel of newspapers. Sunday mornings were especially tough—the papers were thick, and we assembled the advertising sections by hand. This meant starting in the predawn darkness. The satchel wouldn't cut it—Sundays needed the wagon.

Let's just say the wagon was not equipped with snow tires.

I also walked fifteen miles to school, uphill both ways.

Sorry. Couldn't resist.

But seriously, I learned a lot from that job. I had to be on time, or cranky customers would call in complaints. I had to know each customer's preferred drop-off location. Since this was long before online payments were a thing, I had to keep up with billing and collecting subscription fees. It was a lot to handle at eleven, and I'm proud that I did it.

Now, my second job was pretty atypical: I worked at a scuba diving shop. My brother Peter and I were obsessed with getting certified to dive, and we convinced our parents to let us take classes. I built a special rapport with our instructors, who owned the store. Frank was an intimidating former Navy diver who towered well over six feet. His wife, Donna, was likewise an imposing figure—an expert instructor, powerfully athletic, and an astute businesswoman who kept the store humming.

In the decade that followed our certification, scuba diving became a central part of my life. The rest of my brothers and our parents joined in. We had great adventures on family diving vacations that just about made my father broke. I continued my training, gaining advanced certifications. Diving was among the most influential parts of my teenage years, and it's part of what led me to the Coast Guard Academy.

But long before that, I had to learn to wring out a mop.

I started working at the dive store as a teenager, at the youngest age the law allowed.

And I didn't know how to wring out a mop.

And because I didn't wring out the mop very well, I ended up soaking the tile floor of the entrance five minutes before opening time on my first day.

Frank, clearly exasperated, let me know this was not going to fly. He shook his head, muttering that we'd be lucky if no one slipped and broke their skull on my first day. Donna was a little gentler. She smiled and handed me a few towels.

I spent ten minutes on my hands and knees, working to dry the floor with rags, a box fan running. As the parking lot filled up, Frank and Donna made small talk with customers until I got things dry enough to minimize the potential for lawsuits.

After I'd been working there for a year, I was an expert at mopping and quite a bit more confident.

I developed the habit of trying to do two or sometimes even three things at once.

This does not work, because multitasking does not work.

Once, I added an extra zero to a customer's credit card purchase. Her $850 worth of scuba gear instantly became $8,500. The kind woman discovered this only upon the phone message from the fraud department of the credit card company.

This happened because I rang up the purchase while handling a phone call with a different customer.

Frank's voice was deadpan in the after-action debrief: "Do one thing at a time, Paul, and do it right."

Frank and Donna taught me a lot of other stuff over the next few years. I learned about retail and salesmanship. I learned technical skills.

But the most important lessons were more basic.

Simple jobs—like mopping the floor—matter a lot.

Do one thing at a time, and do it well.

Be on time.

When you don't know, ask.

Don't take shortcuts.

Nearly thirty years later, my daily work is far more complex. But those simple lessons are still the most important ones, and I'm grateful for them. Frank and Donna were wonderful mentors to me.

It's the Experience, Not the Pay

There are many reasons to get a job while you're still in high school—or even younger, if you can nab a paper route—and money is probably not the main one. That's not because I'm assuming you are rich. It's because unless you land an unusually lucrative job, the experience is going to be exponentially more valuable than the paycheck. That said, you gain a new appreciation for money when you start trading your free time for it.

Don't be too picky about your first jobs. It isn't about doing something you really enjoy. It's about learning how to work. Of course, if you can find both, then great.

If you're frustrated by the low pay, try this little trick on yourself: just think of your first job as a really good course in life skills—except instead of having to pay for it, you actually get paid a little bit to take the class.

There's another element of the work experience that's really important: the camaraderie of shared labor. I spent a couple years as a busboy (and occasional bartender) at an upscale restaurant in college. The hours were long, and the work was grueling. But you know what? I had a lot of great laughs with the people I worked with. We worked hard, shoulder to shoulder, doing something difficult as part of a team. There were other guys my age, sure. But there were the men and women who'd been at it for a lifetime, too. Servers who showed me what truly excellent customer service looks like. Managers who modeled an amazing level of agility in a stressful, frenetic environment. Dishwashers who showed that even the simplest of work takes endurance and attention to detail—and a hell of a sense of humor.

Looking back, I realize that restaurant work showed me a lot about people and the way we interact. I saw firsthand how horrible people can be—rude customers, for example—and how generous others can be. I saw class-act moments of human kindness and utterly reprehensible behaviors by idiots. The idiots were often trying to impress someone, and usually inspired by one drink too many. I learned how much tips matter to people working in service jobs, and ever since, I've been as generous as I can.

If you're old enough to have a job, then get one, work hard at it, and appreciate it. The experience will give you much more than a paycheck. There is dignity to work. I know it sounds silly to say, "It will make you feel more like a man," but, well, it will make you feel more like a man. That might be enough of a reason by itself.

Oh . . . and you might learn how to wield a mop.

Go ahead. Laugh if you want.

It's harder than you think to do it right.

Jobs, Vocations, and a Career that Blends Both

I have an uncle who once told me the old adage that "if you find a job you love, you'll never work a day in your life." Well, I understand my uncle's good intentions, but the truth is, this is pretty terrible advice, and I wish it weren't so popular among well-intentioned uncles everywhere. If you find a job you love, you'll *absolutely* work hard at it. Hard work and doing something you love aren't mutually exclusive propositions. It's yet another "both/and."

A career, I think, is a blend of two concepts. On one hand, it's a job—but not just *any* job. It's one that fulfills a genuine desire. It responds to a calling. So, on the other hand, it's a vocation. A vocation is, from the Latin root, "a calling." It's the idea that there is something you can do that will bring you fulfillment; a sense of purpose that comes with adding something of meaningful value.

This is in line with our earlier discussion of consolation. Your vocation, if you are fulfilling it, should be a source of consolation. That doesn't mean there won't be some very bad times full of desolation. It just means that if you are generally in a state of consolation with regard to your work, there's a good chance you're living out a vocation.

You'll also notice I said "a vocation," not "*your* vocation."
I've never liked the idea of telling someone to "find your vocation" because it implies that there is just a single, predetermined
path that was somehow picked for you, and if you don't ever
find it, you're somehow missing out on some grandiose cosmic
destiny. To bring us back to the excerpt from Machado's poem
in the opening pages of this book:

> *Caminante, no hay camino,*
> *se hace camino al andar.*
>
> (Walker, there is no road,
> the road is made by walking.)[1]

Building a rewarding career means finding a way to blend
the practical with the inspirational. You need to pay the bills,
but you need to do so in a way that is attentive to your genuine desires. Just because something is a blend of two things, it
doesn't mean the blend is always fifty-fifty. As a general rule,
I think a man should prioritize love of work and fulfillment
over money.

I have talked to guys who have gone down the other road.
They prioritize money over everything else. They figure if
they earn enough, they can tolerate anything. So they bury
themselves in debt to earn a fancy degree from an overpriced
big-name university, then take a prestigious six-figure job that
they quickly come to despise. Then they spend years in a blur

of miserable aimlessness, working sixteen-hour days that leave them drinking hard and crying alone at night in their expensive, lonely big-city condos. Yikes.

But the other extreme can be just as bad. Imagine a musician dedicated to his creative work but struggling with money. He refuses to take a less passionate but better-paying job because he wants his creative freedom. To make matters worse, he claims to be fiscally responsible because he lives simply—yet somehow, he's still constantly in debt anyway. It's not as much debt as guy number one, but it's disproportional to his meager income.

Too much emphasis on the practical at the expense of vocation isn't good, but neither is too much emphasis on the inspirational calling at the expense of the practical.

CONFUSING THE MEANS AND THE ENDS

Too little money can make people unhappy and ruin relationships. No surprise, right? Of course, so can too much money. If you know any miserable rich people, you already know this. Somewhere, there seems to be a tipping point—a point of diminishing returns on income, when earning more stops making you happier.

It's hard to believe this point exists if you are far from hitting it, wherever it may be. If you're still in high school, for example, this might not seem too relevant. If you're right out of college in the first few years of your career, making too much money is probably *not* a problem you'll have to deal with anytime soon.

But I would assert that the point of diminishing returns *is* there for each of us, and if we aren't paying attention, we can move right past it while we're working hard to climb. After a while, though, we'll realize something has changed.

Where it gets tricky is determining where that tipping point lies. There's been research that claims to have identified it. For example, a widely cited 2010 Princeton study[2] found that it was $75,000 for an individual, which is roughly $107,000 in 2024 dollars, adjusted for inflation. But then, more recently, a 2021 study from Penn[3] refuted that assertion, suggesting that people continued to get happier as they made more money. Interestingly, the researchers behind these two studies later got together to reconcile their findings, which seemed to be at odds. Their conclusion, basically, was that people who are *already happy* tend to keep getting happier with more money, whereas people who are *already unhappy* see their happiness increases plateau after a hundred thousand dollars.[4]

So, who knows, really? There are many variables and assumptions built into any theory like this. Much would depend on lifestyle, cost of living, and other incomes in the household. Ultimately, it seems to me that the relationship between money and happiness would depend on the person, which is of course what the latest study suggests. It's no surprise that there are greater underlying determinators of happiness than money, and if those factors are suffering, more money can only do so much to improve happiness or quality of life—or the relationships at the core of both.

Sometimes we can get confused about the means and the ends. If you can think of money as a *means* to higher end purposes—your family, your responsibilities, and, ultimately, your telos—you'll be able to keep things in perspective and avoid tipping the balance. But if you get that confused, and you begin thinking of money as the end itself, well, you're in for a world of hurt. Work hard and earn money—lots, if you can.

Just don't confuse the means with the ends.

A Basic Principle of Economics

If you want to make intelligent decisions about work, money, and freedom, you need to understand a very basic principle of economics: Nothing is without cost. Actually, this relates to two basic laws of physics. The Principle of Mass Conservation tells us that matter cannot be created or destroyed, only transformed. Similarly, the First Law of Thermodynamics states that energy cannot be created or destroyed; it can only be transmitted or otherwise transformed. So, in that sense, everything comes at a cost. Even the air we breathe comes at a cost—it requires the chemical process that generates the breathable compounds of nitrogen and oxygen, which comprise all but a tiny percentage of what we breathe.

This applies to finances, too. If you go to college on a full scholarship, that doesn't mean that your education is "free." It may, from where you stand, come without a financial cost, but it is certainly not free. Someone has paid, is paying, or will pay for it, whether through debt, taxes, tuition grants, subsidies, or scholarship endowments, whatever the case may be. Nothing is without cost. Of course, that's a good thing. Because if you have even the most rudimentary understanding of economics, you know that something without cost would, effectively, have no value. Value is interconnected with cost.

This applies both in financial and nonfinancial terms. When it comes to money, that new tablet you want has value, which is reflected in its price tag—and vice versa. Likewise, a meaningful relationship has value, but it also has a cost commensurate with its value. It demands things like time, effort, patience, investment, sacrifice, and love. Of course, if you know about another basic principle of economics, you know that supply and demand are inversely related—when the supply of something exceeds the demand for it, the value of that thing goes down—and so does its cost. Conversely, when the demand for something is disproportionate to the available supply, the value is higher—as is the cost. We saw this during the pandemic, for example, when low demand for gas and diesel during the shutdowns of 2020 created a massive oversupply and sent the price of crude oil plummeting. On the flip side (and somewhat ironically), the prices of cars skyrocketed due to high demand and reduced supply.

Okay. So, scarcity can boost value, and oversupply diminishes value. This may seem obvious in terms of money—but if you really want to understand the "economics" of a balanced life, you have to look at costs beyond the financial ones.

Opportunity Costs

Let's say you're a teenage lifeguard and you work at a local athletic center for fifteen dollars an hour. You made plans to see a movie with your friends on Friday night. You've been looking forward to it all week. Just as you're getting ready, the manager calls you and tells you she's short lifeguards for four hours that evening. She's really desperate, and she offers you thirty dollars an hour if you'll cover it. Double your normal pay rate. Do you give up going out with your friends and pick up an extra $120 instead of spending money on the movie? Tough call, right?

Gets tougher later in life, when the stakes are higher. I started a small consulting business in my late twenties. At first, it was just a little bit of tutoring, along with editing some book manuscripts and helping people fine-tune their resumés. I ended up landing a few corporate clients, and the business grew to become a second job that I did outside the confines of the school day. Eventually, it grew enough that I dialed teaching down to part-time so I could continue to build the consulting work. It's tough work, but fascinating—and it really changed my family's financial picture.

But opportunity cost is a real thing. Here's an example. It was a beautiful Saturday afternoon in autumn. My kids were excited for a bike ride and backyard campout. We were just checking the bike tires when I got an email from a client about a last-minute writing project. It was a sweet deal if I wanted it, but it would have to be done immediately—as in, by 11:59 that night.

I knew the kids would be disappointed, but the six-hour job would pay *a lot*. By "a lot," I mean more than I used to make in a whole week of teaching. No brainer, right? That time, I chose the job. The kids were let down, but I promised them a bike ride and backyard campout the following weekend.

This happening once or twice is not that big a deal. Here's the thing, though—you might be surprised how frequently this type of dilemma arises as you grow older, no matter how much you earn and what field you work in.

Whether it's an extra lifeguarding shift or a lucrative corporate contract, the danger is the same: It can become a pattern of opportunity costs. Mutually exclusive opportunities will present themselves.

You have to pay attention to your patterns, because the more this happens, the harder it gets to prioritize relationships over income. It may not sound like much of a trap, but it can become one. The collateral damage can be heavy. Relationships can suffer. Ruining that Saturday evening with my kids *once* wasn't the end of the world.

The real challenge came the following weekend, when I'd promised to make up the bike ride and camp out. Because guess what happened? Yep. You know it. Another last-minute job—and just as lucrative. I turned it down that time, and we had a great afternoon as a family. Now, I wish I could tell you I didn't even have to think twice about it. I did. But I've learned it's not singular choices that define us. It's our patterns that define us. Our patterns reveal our priorities.

Your Greatest Financial Asset: Time

I bet you've often been told you should save money. If you're like most young guys, that doesn't really register on the level that it should. This is because it often isn't explained very well, in school or anywhere else. We're *told* to save our pennies, but we aren't really *shown* why, using math.

Do you know what your greatest financial asset is? It's not your family's net worth. It's not your job. It's not your education or your fancy college degree. It's not your ambition or your drive or your work ethic. It's your youth. Yeah, that's right. It's time.

Math has never been my strong suit, but I understand compounding interest. When you have a set amount of money ("principal") and you apply a percentage multiplier ("interest rate") to it repeatedly, on a periodic basis, you create a situation where not only does the amount increase over time, but the *rate* at which the amount increases also increases.

The younger you are at the beginning of the compounding equation, the more time there is for the compounding to happen. In other words, each dollar you put in at age eighteen will, in the long run, be worth considerably more than each dollar you put in at twenty-five.

The younger you are, the greater the advantage. Conversely, the older you get, the more quickly that advantage decreases. All of this, by the way, is without even addressing the various tax advantages that come with this type of long-term savings.

Obviously, there are limits to this. If you're focused so heavily on saving maximally for later and costing yourself important opportunities now, you're maybe taking it too far. You've gotta live, man. But most people have the opposite problem, and don't save enough when they're young.

I'll use myself as an example. I looked at my retirement balances recently, along with my savings history. I realized that it wasn't until age twenty-five that I really began ramping up my long-term retirement savings. I wondered how much difference it would have made if I'd saved more at twenty-two, twenty-three, and twenty-four. I used a compounding calculator (you can find them online) and I figured out that if I had saved just $1,500 more for each of those years, the difference would likely be close to $60,000 by the time I retire.

This made me wince as I recalled the cutting-edge twenty-seven-inch, 720p flatscreen I just *had* to have when I was twenty-three. It was about fifteen hundred dollars. Ouch.

Starting your disciplined savings at twenty-two instead of twenty-five makes a big difference. No matter what age you are, find out how to take advantage of your biggest financial asset: time. This book is not focused on financial literacy, so it's not my intention to get into the weeds on this stuff. But, if you want to get started learning more about this, I suggest taking a little time to learn about just two basic terms.

First, search up "retirement calculator" and play around with some numbers. Second, learn what a Roth IRA is. If you're earning a paycheck, you can probably open one—and you should. If you start by learning about just those two topics, you'll get a jump on understanding how to invest for long-term wealth. Finally, if you're employed, talk to whoever manages human resources or payroll and find out what options exist to maximize the power of your savings. You might be surprised to learn that your company may have policies in place that can help you save more—or might even contribute to your long-term savings.

CHARITY ON THE PATH

I can't finish this chapter without connecting it with the previous one on service. One of the greatest gifts that comes with accumulating some money is the ability to give it away.

Yeah, you read that right.

I can think of many times in my life when I've been the recipient of someone else's financial generosity. And here I'm not talking about anything earned or deserved. I'm talking about someone's generosity, plain and simple.

When I consider the scholarships that helped defray my high school and college tuition bills, I know that came from someone who'd decided to put their money into the service of those schools.

When I think about the mentors who have helped me get my businesses off the ground, I know I want to be able to do the same someday for someone else. Charitable generosity is one of the "ends" that money affords.

232

It certainly isn't the only form of service by a long shot, but it is a powerful thing indeed to be able to help people through generosity. And in the same way that savings can compound, so too can charity. Because charity tends to beget charity. In my experience, people tend to "pay it forward" in one way or another.

That's a nice pattern, for sure.

——

There's a story I made up years ago that I use to teach freshmen about irony in literature. It goes like this.

Once upon a time there was a high school kid named Mark. Several months earlier, he'd met a girl named Emily, and they'd really hit it off. They'd been dating ever since.

At one point while they were walking through the mall, Emily noticed a designer coat that she really loved. When she looked at the price tag, she laughed and shook her head.

Mark knew her birthday was in a month and a half. As he noticed Emily checking out pictures of the same coat online later that afternoon, he made up his mind to get it for her. The coat wasn't cheap, but it wasn't too much. He already had his monthly car payment and his smartphone bill, though, so Mark knew he'd have to push.

He redoubled his hours at the pizza shop where he worked after school and on weekends. He took on extra shifts for several weekends in a row. He began to see Emily less often.

When he did, she sometimes seemed distracted. Something felt different, and Mark figured it was that he'd been so busy with work—but he knew it was worth it. Just a couple more weeks, he told himself.

Finally, a week before Emily's birthday, Mark headed to the mall, cash in hand. He picked up the jacket in her size and had it professionally gift wrapped.

When he got home, Emily texted him. She asked if they could meet up over coffee and talk. As they sat on a park bench, steaming cups of coffee in their hands, she began to cry as she told him it seemed like maybe they needed some time apart.

Hating to ruin the surprise but knowing he needed to explain, Mark told Emily the whole story, and he smiled as he gave her the birthday present right there in the park.

She was surprised and thrilled, of course, but she told Mark how much it had hurt when she thought he was giving her the cold shoulder.

Mark shook his head, feeling like an idiot. It was true, he realized. In his relentless push to earn money for the gift, he'd been ignoring the relationship itself.

That's irony.

He apologized, and it all ended well. Emily put on the new coat. They went for a walk around the park, hand in hand. They laughed every time they told the story to their friends.

When it comes to work, money, and freedom, don't confuse the means and the ends.

Keep relationships at the heart of your decisions.

Your patterns reveal your priorities.

CHAPTER SIXTEEN

Hearts and Rings

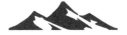

My wife's grandfather was a high school math teacher and father of seven. As the story goes, a friend of his once made a remark to him that because this friend only had two children, he only had to divide his love *two* ways, whereas a father of seven had to divide his love *seven* ways, to the disadvantage of each. My grandfather-in-law corrected the man, explaining that he had the math wrong, and that it didn't work that way.

But you don't have to be a math teacher to understand that of course it doesn't work that way. The equation of love does not work on zero-sum terms.

A parent does not proportionally dole out diminishing portions of love as the number of children increases. Rather, the love compounds upon itself, like a cloud billowing and expanding. This is not to say that the father of seven has "more" love than the father of two; no, that would be working on the same flawed calculus.

When we love, the equations go out the window. It isn't a rational, logical thing. We can't account for it. Accounting doesn't work well in relationships.

It isn't a transaction or an arrangement.

It's companionship.

Love Is Not a Zero-Sum Equation

We tend to approach everything in a transactional way, which is natural. After all, our very survival depends upon transactions. We kill or harvest to eat. We sleep in order to wake. When we are wronged, our instinct is vengeance—even if we manage not to act on it. We return kindness for kindness.

If you always remember your friend's birthday, but they never remember yours, it hurts—if only a little bit, maybe—because it isn't fair. Almost all of life runs on the economics of transaction. As we discussed earlier, nothing is entirely without cost.

But love—genuine love—doesn't work by the same calculus as most things. There is certainly a cost to love, no doubt about it. It requires sacrifices of all kinds. A real friendship, let alone a healthy marriage, is not a zero-sum proposition; that is, it is not transactional by design. It isn't a fifty-fifty arrangement. It isn't always "fair." It doesn't always "equal out."

Ask anyone who's been married for even just a few years. If you want everything to be equal and fair all the time, you're destined for disappointment, because you're looking at it wrong. Both parties have to be willing to give more than they take.

If that sounds like weird math, it is.

That's love.

Obviously, if both parties give more than they take, this does not work out to anything resembling transactional equality, and it doesn't add up to some kind of relational 100 percent. Here's the thing: if you expect it to, your expectations are going to be problematic.

But here's the other thing: Even if we know a relationship is not always going to be "fair," for some reason, we still expect it to be. Because that's natural. Because we're human, and we're more or less selfish.

And that's why genuinely loving relationships are hard. They cost a lot. They're supposed to. Why should we expect anything of value not to? The good news is, as the story about my wife's grandfather taught me, love works by its own calculus. It's beyond exponential.

TEENAGE RELATIONSHIPS

When we're young, say, in high school, which is when most of us are first trying out intimate relationships like having a "significant other," this transactional thing is very apparent.

I ask you to my prom; you ask me to yours. I venture into this level of intimacy with you; you with me. I gain the social capital and self-affirmation that comes with having you as my significant other; you gain all of the same in return.

Generally, the relationship goes well as long as the transactional record is fairly even. This is not to say the relationships of youth are cheap or insignificant. Not at all. I think it's fair to say that with each party's respective future stretching out before them, there's little sense that either owes the other any sort of massively consequential investment.

In fact, that's precisely what allows you the freedom to experiment with increasingly "committed" relationships—the fact that they're not, in fact, committing you, as in locking you in. After all, it's prom, dude, not marriage. Even the most intense high school relationships tend to end—or at least go on a lengthy hiatus—after high school, because, well, it's time for them to end, and both parties know this deep down, even if they don't like it.

And yet taking the risk to embark on these often-messy forays into deepening relationships is so important. It is this experimentation with love that allows you to begin to understand your emotional capacity. It compels you to develop an emotional vocabulary. You realize the challenge and beauty of intimacy, both emotional and, in many cases, physical. You have experiences that make clear just how powerful the movements of the heart can be, and how readily they can knock you off your feet.

You come to grips with yourself as a sexual being (hopefully gradually) and get a sense of what powerful forces get unleashed in that context. You experience your feelings with an acute sensitivity more refined than that of a child—that means new depths of emotional lows along with newfound, stratospheric highs.

The magnitude of this emotional pendulum swinging from despair to joy, along with the added momentum of your emerging sexual drives, can certainly get you in a heap of trouble. However, it can also teach you things you need to know about being human.

The thing to remember about intimate relationships at a young age is that they are all about companionship on a *part* of the camino, the path. As intense as your companionship at this stage may be, your ways are all but certain to diverge, and that's okay. If you treat each other as companions who will someday travel separate paths, you can journey together in peace without unrealistic expectations.

But along with tempering those expectations—and I think this is tricky for teenagers in serious relationships—it's important to temper your behaviors, too. Making sense of sexual feelings and attractions can sometimes be confusing, so be patient with yourself as you navigate this part of your path. My suggestion is, err on the side of slowing down. It's not a race. You don't need to prove yourself to anyone—including yourself—by doing something you're not ready to do. If you don't realistically expect to have a lifelong commitment to each other, then you better be pretty damn careful about how physically intimate you become. There are good reasons why very old faith traditions forbid sex before marriage. Maybe you think it's all just about stodgy, outdated, archaic value systems. Nope, sorry man, but it's really pretty rational. Because until you're locked into a mutual commitment, it's very risky to do things that potentially get you, well, locked into a mutual commitment.

On the most obvious, physiological level (in a heterosexual relationship), that might mean pregnancy. As a husband and father, I cannot even *begin to try* to convey to anyone who is not a parent the magnitude and gravity of what pregnancy means. To truly even begin to convey this would take another book unto itself—and is not one any man could write, in my opinion. Only a woman could write that book.

Beyond the question of pregnancy, there are other physical issues, such as sexually transmitted infections. But beyond these physical considerations lies something I think teenagers often fail to understand: the emotional and psychological weight of sexual intimacy, no matter with whom. Don't underestimate that. It isn't a "casual thing." The morning after can suddenly get very real, very quickly, and I don't just mean physical consequences. Sexual experimentation isn't exactly uncommon among teenagers, but just because something is typical doesn't mean it should be taken lightly. Getting physically intimate with someone is, well, a genie you can't put back in the bottle.

Companionship in your teenage years is so important, and an intimate relationship can help you begin to understand the beauty and complexity of life in ways you'll need to as an adult. Just remember that your companions at that age, no matter how intimate they may become, are likely to travel with you only for a while. Don't jeopardize the rest of the journey for either traveler. That's a matter of respect—for oneself and for the other.

BACHELOR RELATIONSHIPS

Things get more complicated later on. Most people agree that the teenage years are not the ideal time to consider delving into a serious, long-term relationship—so the expectations tend to be low, and, with the exception of rare situations, so do the consequences of messing up. Plenty of teenagers stub their toes as they navigate relationships, but compared to the treacherous terrain facing guys in, say, their twenties, it tends to be a reasonably safe section of the path.

Enter young adulthood, and the camino gets rockier. Stakes get higher, and so do expectations. When it comes to young adults navigating "serious" relationships, there are all sorts of pitfalls and traps. Here are three traps I've seen a lot of guys fall into:

Trap 1: Fearlessly rushing in

Trap 2: Fearfully rushing in

Trap 3: Fear of commitment

We'll take a look at those first, and then I'll share what I think is a key to success in bachelor relationships.

TRAP 1: FEARLESSLY RUSHING IN

Let's talk about trap 1: fearlessly rushing in. This tends to be the province of younger guys—the overgrown teenager types—who can often be immature fools, motivated and driven more by ego and libido than anything resembling wisdom. What I mean by having no fear is having no mature appreciation for what's at stake in a relationship. This can be due to ignorance, naïveté, carelessness, or some combination of these. When it's out of carelessness, it's easy to call it reckless and selfish. When it's due more to youthful ignorance or naïveté, it tends to seem less malicious, but it's still dangerous. Regardless of the reason, here's what it usually looks like: Playing fast and loose with powerful forces and emotions. Taking a cavalier approach to relationships, almost as though they are some sort of sport, or trophies to be put on display. Underestimating—or worse yet, disregarding—the potential for serious harm and lasting ill effects. In other words, playing the role of the proverbial bull in the china shop in terms of people's feelings and well-being. For a lot of guys, the most obvious manifestation of this is careless sexual activity, with little regard for physiological, psychological, and emotional implications.

TRAP 2: FEARFULLY RUSHING IN

Trap 2, rushing in out of fear, is different. It may seem similar to trap 1, since it certainly sounds like a case of reckless immaturity, but let me make a distinction. I would posit that some pretty mature guys find themselves in danger of trap 2. These might be hardworking, level-headed young men. They might be diligent and conscientious. They often have many boxes checked: good education? Check. Steady job and career focus? Check. Reasonably balanced, well-adjusted, and in good health? Check. At the same time, they might also be scared to death of the one box that remains conspicuously *un*checked: solid relationship.

Oh, yeah. This one's trouble for many guys. Big trouble, because it revolves around insecurity and social pressure. Not just peer pressure, either. Nope—this one's got the added bonus of family and societal pressure. This can come across in many ways. *When are you going to settle down? Gosh, you're so well adjusted. What's the missing link? Are you afraid of commitment? You know, you're not getting any younger. What, is no one good enough for you? So many of your friends are engaged. I just wish you could find the right person so you could be happy.*

So, that sets the stage for trap 2, rushing in out of fear. Take a guy in his late twenties, for example. He's been in and out of a number of relationships. None have really worked out. This latest relationship, though? It's pretty good. In fact, it seems really solid. He's not 100 percent sure, but who can be 100 percent sure about anything, really? If he's not sure he's in love, well, maybe if he just commits, he'll find his way there. Right? And man, either way, it really seems like it's about time he get himself hitched.

What does he do? He commits out of fear. It has more to do with calming his own insecurities than it does with genuine love. Before long, he buys a ring. He gets engaged, often to the cheers, joy, and even relief of family and friends. It can all seem very mature and responsible and "on the right track." Yet, if it was motivated primarily out of fear—out of insecurity, really— why should he expect it to work? It might. On the other hand, it very well might not, and that's a high-stakes gamble, motivated mostly by self-interest. A decision made principally out of fear—particularly more or less selfish fear like this—is generally not a well-discerned decision.

Trap 3: Fear of Commitment

A lot of guys spend years looking for the "perfect match."

Sometimes it's misplaced effort. There's nothing wrong with searching for the "right" person, but searching for the "perfect" person is probably going to involve lots of time, frustration, and tears. Romantic literature and movies convince us that fate and love are somehow intertwined. That by default, there *is* some ideal person out there, just waiting for a complex arrangement of cosmic circumstances to align properly for us to meet.

Consider how many of us believe this, even though we don't believe in fate when it comes to other parts of our lives. When an aspiring professional athlete experiences a life-altering injury that destroys his dreams, ask him if it was fate. He'll first probably tell you to shut the hell up, and then quickly add that no, it wasn't fate, it was a split-second wrong move or an arbitrary random collision.

Ask a happily employed guy if he thinks it was his fate to work at this particular company, and he'll look at you funny and say, "No, man, I *worked* my way here."

But ask a guy if he thinks it was fate that connected him with the particular woman who is now his wife and the mother of his children, and he'll get smoke in his eyes and nod sagaciously, as though he's been let in on one of the great cosmic mysteries of life. As though, no matter how many missteps he made, sooner or later he was *bound* to meet this specific woman and live this specific life.

Maybe fate's a thing and maybe it isn't. I don't know.

What I *can* tell you is that when you squander a genuinely loving relationship because you're holding out for someone "better" or even "perfect," be careful. Fear of commitment can take on many disguises. Among the most common is "holding out for something better." Well, maybe that's wise, up to a point. But only up to a point.

EVERYTHING BUT MARRIAGE?

A lot of loud voices in our culture have proclaimed that marriage is an outdated social construct. That it has outlived its usefulness. I couldn't disagree more. We need more marriage, not less. I'll acknowledge that marriage isn't the right path for everyone. I'll also acknowledge that it is an extraordinarily difficult undertaking. But that doesn't negate its value—in fact, I'd say the difficulty is part of its value proposition. I suspect there are many people whose lives would be deeply enriched by marriage if they weren't ideologically convinced that it wasn't for them.

Imagine a guy and his girlfriend, both in their late twenties. They've been dating for years. They're obviously in love and deeply committed to one another. This isn't a passing relationship. They're sexually intimate, of course. They've moved in together. They even share a joint bank account to manage their rent, groceries, utilities, and other shared expenses. They raise a puppy together. Their respective families each adore the other. They are both convinced they'll be married.

But here's the kicker: "Just not yet."

If we were to ask this guy what the hell the two of them are waiting for, the response is likely to be a series of mumbled, noncommittal half-assertions about the time not being right, about just wanting to finish paying off student loans, and waiting until something or the other is "situated."

I've had essentially this same conversation with a number of guys over the past ten years—former students who have come to me for advice, knowing I'm happily married with kids. Obviously, the circumstances have varied. But more or less, that's the story. And each time, without trying to push too hard in one direction or the other, I've asked the same question: "Well man, what's the difference between how you're living and how you'd be living if you were married?"

And each time, it's been pretty hard to come up with a difference.

"Except that you'd be locked in," I suggest.

"Yeah. I guess I just don't know if we're ready for that," has been the reply.

Hmm. Genuinely in love. Living together. Sleeping together. Joint bank accounts. Families in love. Planning on marriage. Yet, somehow, not ready to commit to one another.

What more does it take? What more should a couple expect? Some kind of cosmic guarantee that it's going to work out? A magic insurance agent who can assure elimination of all risk?

This is trap 3 at the most critical level: everything in place for a *truly* committed relationship, except for the final piece— the *actual* commitment.

That commitment of marriage might feel like a "trap," but it's actually the very thing that will set the relationship free. If, that is—and man, this is an *extraordinarily* important if— it is genuinely grounded in mature love. The kind of love that isn't transactional. The kind of love that isn't looking for fifty-fifty. The kind of love that doesn't need (or even want) a prenuptial agreement. If that's truly the case, and it is real love, then "locking in" the relationship is, paradoxically, the key to ultimate freedom.

All of this may make sense in one's rational, analytical mind. So why the common hesitation? Simple. It's fear. Fear of being wrong. Fear of it not being perfect. Fear of it not working out.

Fear, fear, fear.

If you think I'm being cavalier or dismissive about fear, let me set the record straight. I know all about fear. I'm a dad—that should tell you enough. But I'll go further. As a married guy, I can tell you that marriage—the true, lifelong commitment, the *contract before God* that says "you and me forever"—is *absolutely terrifying*. Do you think it has ever been any different, though? Do you think all the billions of men who came before us and got married didn't face the same fear? Of course it's terrifying. How could it not be? You're *locking in*, man! And yes, it could fail!

But guess what? It's also the greatest antidote to that fear. How can that be? How can something be both the cause of fear and antidote to it? Well, think about it. That's pretty much *always* the case. If you're scared of the dark, you become less scared of the dark by spending time in the dark. If you're terrified of spiders, you gradually acclimatize yourself to the presence of spiders. When you were learning to drive and you were terrified about merging into freeway traffic, you only got over it by . . . wait for it . . . merging into freeway traffic.

It's like that in marriage, but you get a huge advantage—a copilot who's committed to being with you. You acknowledge the reality of those fears *together*. You enter willingly into a situation that you both know hinges entirely on the *two* of you. You *both* fully commit, knowing the whole thing rests on each other's strengths *and* human imperfections. That's an act of tremendous faith. It's a *mutual* act of faith.

It's hard. But there is great freedom in it.

In part, because it has the power to change the nature of your fears.

Let me explain that. I had a conversation not too long ago with a group of guys in their twenties attending one of our young men's trips in the Dominican Republic. One of them asked me if I liked being a middle-aged dad. I told him I love it, despite the slower metabolism, dad bod, and receding hairline. When he asked why, I told him this: I'm not afraid anymore. Then, after a pause, I clarified that statement. I told him that of course I still have fears, but I'm at the stage in my life where my fears very rarely have anything to do with myself anymore. My most genuine fears are all about others—my wife and my kids.

Committing your life to someone else can be a great anti-dote to at least one kind of fear—the existential fears you have about yourself. Because when your life becomes about someone else, you just don't have as much time for that stuff anymore.

A Key to Success

Okay, so those are three traps, along with some thoughts about marriage. But I mentioned I'd also share a "key to success." Notice I said *a* key to success, not *the* key to success. I'm not saying it's the *only* key to success. I just happen to believe it's a pretty reliable one:

Love and embrace the truth.

Sounds simple enough, but like I mentioned earlier in the book using the example of digging a hole in the ground, something can be very simple and also very difficult. Loving the truth means genuinely desiring to be true in a relationship. That means being honest. It means telling the truth, of course, but it also means *being* true. Not holding back the truth and trying to put forth what you think the one you love *wants* to hear. Because you won't be able to sustain that.

Think of it this way. In marriage, you have to be willing to be fully naked before the one you love. Consider physical nakedness as a metaphor here. You have to be willing to be naked, with all the lights on, with all of your most flattering—and unflattering—aspects in full view. You have to do so with the knowledge that you can't just run out the door if you don't like what you see—and neither can the person you've committed to. You can't hide things—at least not sustainably, so why bother? Just imagine for a moment how simultaneously scary *and* affirming that is! That's loving and embracing the truth.

If you're in a relationship and hiding from the other person, only showing that person the parts of you that you want seen, that isn't loving the truth. It's sure as hell not embracing it.

See, loving isn't just "liking a lot." Loving is embracing and taking care of things, even things you don't like. Got problems, weaknesses, and iniquities? You've got to *love* them, man, even if you despise them. The person you're marrying—that person also has problems, weaknesses, and iniquities. You have to *love* those aspects, even if you don't like them. That's loving the truth—the truth about who we are. The whole, human package. Not just the shiny stuff.

That doesn't mean you can't change or shouldn't try. No! Loving a problem can definitely involve changing it—in fact, it probably *has to* involve trying to change it. That's why I suggested it's better to think of loving as "taking care of and working on" rather than just a stronger form of "liking" something. When you define love that way, you realize that when it comes to dealing with a problem or weakness—whether your own or on the part of someone you love—you have to love the problem or weakness first. Because *like* it or not, the problem or weakness is part of the person.

Why are rings the symbol of marriage? It's traditionally because they represent an infinite commitment—no beginning or end. Know what else? The circle is a *strong* structure. It is remarkably good at withstanding pressure, whether from the outside pushing in or the inside pushing out. It redistributes force quite effectively. Taken three-dimensionally, we see this in the shape of the deepest-diving submarines, the cylindrical construction of water towers and grain elevators, and the circular convergence of the world's largest domed cathedrals.

Commitment demands a lot, but it makes you stronger. Take your time, and don't rush things. But when you're old enough, when the time is right, and most importantly when the love is real, don't let fear of commitment get in the way. Because there's no greater gift than lifelong companionship— mutually committed, for better or for worse, in sickness or in health—when it comes to traveling your path.

CHAPTER SEVENTEEN

A Case for Faith

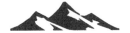

IF YOU'VE EVER BEEN around a group of guys building a campfire, you know what always happens. One claims to be the expert in the log cabin method. Another dude shouts him down, clamoring for the teepee design. Some clown just wants to douse it in gasoline. A well-meaning helper doesn't know any better and throws on a thick log too soon, extinguishing it, and everyone groans.

After lots of arguing, the quiet guy who actually knows what the hell he's doing gets the thing started. A solemn hush descends as the rest stand around with hands shoved in their pockets and serious expressions on their faces, their manly presence *willing* the fire to grow.

It takes a while to build a good fire. One hastily built will burn brightly for a minute or two, but it won't withstand the wind. It'll be a show of big flames with nothing at the heart. Lots of light; very little heat.

The heart of the fire is the key. It takes patient nurturing for those coals to burn with the subtle red glow of sustained heat. That's what faith is like. Faith is the heart of the fire.

No Assumptions

I purposely put this chapter last, because I've tried to write this book the same way I try to teach: show first; tell second.

Let me put it another way. If you wanted to explain inertia and momentum to a young kid, you'd be better off letting him play with a set of marbles first. Or, if you wanted to discuss how to write a short story, you start by reading a well-written story or two.

When teachers approach complex topics in this way—before explaining the terms, theories, concepts, and forces themselves—then you have an experiential basis. That's why, for the most part, I've resisted infusing too much theological or religious language into the previous chapters. I wanted to *show* you what my faith means to me in everyday life before *telling* you in religious terms.

I didn't want to assume religious faith on your part. I still don't. But since you've read this far, you are a "thinking being" of the type Saint Paul called the Romans to be. So let me offer you a couple thoughts about faith and religion.

What Does It Mean to Be Religious?

Words can tell us a lot. "Religion" traces to Latin *religare*, which translates "to bind fast," as in "to adhere strongly." By this logic, to be religious means to adhere to something—a belief, a set of principles, or perhaps a practice.

When a student tells me he's not religious, he usually means that he doesn't consider himself part of an institutional religion—call it a "capital 'R' religion."

But I sometimes push back and suggest maybe he's religious with a small "r." I challenge him to think about his devotion to his academic work, or his athletic pursuits, or his disciplined commitment to taking care of his baby sister.

To be religious means to bind oneself to something of meaning. The world's "capital 'R' religions" are frameworks—usually ancient ones—of commitment. They are a guidebook for how to make your path, bound to certain principles.

And generally, in the pursuit of virtue.

I think a lot of guys are religious, even if they don't think they are. Even if they have all kinds of doubts and questions.

FAITH DESPITE THE MESS

A lot of people, of all ages, struggle with their faith on multiple levels. In some cases, this involves mistrust of religious institutions—and often for quite understandable reasons. In other cases, it might be a matter of skepticism about the very existence of God. I get it. As someone raised in the Roman Catholic Church, and furthermore as someone who has spent his entire career to date working in Catholic schools, I am in some ways deeply disillusioned and disappointed in the failings of the institutional Church that have come to light in recent decades.

Following my younger brother's wedding, I wrote an op-ed for our city newspaper. I'll share it with you here, because I think it helps to articulate how and why I remain a person of faith despite that very real disillusionment and disappointment.

My brother got married last weekend. As he and his wife professed their vows, I felt genuine joy and a sense that things were as they ought to be. Our family is Catholic, so this joy emerged despite troubled times. In fact, just hours after the wedding, an interview aired in which our pastor called publicly for the bishop's resignation.

My four brothers and I attended the same Catholic elementary school and Jesuit high school. We were all altar servers. We are all married in the Church. To my knowledge, across more than a cumulative half-century of Catholic education, none of us was abused. Church was not always where we wanted to be on Sunday morning, but it mattered. Catholicism shaped our moral development, setting clear rules and offering redemption when we messed up. It was a backdrop for childhood. Christmas. Easter. Weddings. Funerals. Brunch at Grandma's.

The crisis hits close to home, then—not explicitly for us, but existentially.

My brothers—all local—work in medicine, information technology, media production, and digital animation. For twenty-two years, I've either coached or taught at Jesuit high schools, working alongside many good Jesuit priests and brothers—virtuous men and servant-leaders. The spirituality of Saint Ignatius Loyola, founder of the Jesuits, invites us to deeper relationships with ourselves, others, and God through honest discernment of our most authentic desires. That has helped me to look deeper, beyond the occasional impulse to cut, run, and slam the door on the whole institution.

But I haven't been going to church much. Is that a failure? A response? A nonresponse? I don't know. Maybe all of the above. Mass was always a "joyful burden," but Sundays now come with a dose of resentment for having committed to an institution that has been negligently and even criminally mismanaged at some levels. To be honest, a morning of blueberry pancakes and cartoons with my wife and kids has, lately, felt more sacramental.

So, a lot churned through my mind and heart at the wedding. But somewhere in there, through what I think is called grace, our broken church embraced me again. Because of family. Our family's strength—suddenly compounded by marriage— was tangible. Our little kids and their great-grandparents were bound together in kairos, *which is Greek for "an opportune time." C. S. Lewis called* kairos *a "decisive, momentary unveiling of the eternal."*

That's why, as my grandmother looked on, I knew my grandfather was with us, holding hands with his bride, to whom he made those same timeless vows nearly a century ago. We buried him a few years ago, but the sureness that he has not ceased to exist is grounded in our shared faith. We are more than material stuff—we are eternal children of God. Saint Paul's letter to the Corinthians reminded us that

love "bears all things, believes all things, hopes all things, and
endures all things." Love is the very nature of Christ. Love
and family, then, are intertwined with God.

No, my kairos *moment does not reconcile the brokenness of*
our church. It does not diminish the crimes, the rank offenses, the
very antitheses of Christian love that such abuses comprise. It
does not excuse mendacity. But it does affirm that our Church
is bigger and stronger than its weakest, most horrific parts.

I'll go to Mass amid the mess. I support calls for change—
including changes in leadership for which many good priests
have called. Deep in my heart, I'll hold to the truths our
church and family have taught my brothers and me since we
were little. Because in those truths lie faith, hope, and love. If
those are not the keys to the redemption of our church, I don't
know what possibly could be.[1]

In that column, I tried to distinguish the failings of a system
from the *complete* failure of that system. That isn't willful ignorance. It's nuanced discernment. Thus, despite my disappoint-
ments, which are real and acute, my faith remains strong. Since
the restrictions in place from the pandemic have eased, my wife
and I have made efforts to take our kids to Mass each week, and
to make religious education a part of their lives.

In Saint Paul's letter to the Romans, he wrote "Think of
God's mercy, my brothers, and worship Him, I beg you, in
a manner worthy of thinking beings" (Romans 12:1–2). I'm
grateful for the privilege of a religious education that has challenged me to think critically about my beliefs.

"A Thrill of Hope"

Here's the first thing I believe because of my Catholic faith. I believe each person is an intentionally created child of a loving God. The Gospel message of Jesus Christ is predicated upon this core principle. To me, it is the foundation for the ultimate telos—that our ultimate destiny is eternal union with God. Crucial to that is the belief that we all matter intensely and deeply and powerfully to God. We are loved not despite our humanity, but indeed *because* of it. That's the core of the Christmas story, right? God chose to manifest as the God-Man, Jesus, whose entry into the world was about as humble and human as you can get.

I find a wonderful articulation of this faith tradition in the classic Christmas song, "O Holy Night," which is based on a translation of a nineteenth-century poem called "Minuit, Chrétiens" (Midnight, Christians) by Placide Cappeau. To me, this song, the music of which was composed by another Frenchman, Adolphe Adam, is among the best expressions of faith and the profound optimism that underlies Christianity. Part of why I think it works so well is that it merges three things essential to Christian tradition. Consider these lines:

> Long lay the world in sin and error pining,
> Till He appear'd and the soul felt its worth.
> A thrill of hope, the weary world rejoices,
> For yonder breaks a new and glorious morn.[2]

First, there's an acknowledgment of what a mess we all are. Then, with that understood, there's the assertion that we matter in a profound and real way—at the level of our souls. Third, there's that bit about hope and a brighter future.

The second verse goes on to convey the essential paradox of the lowly king, the God-child—the unlikely embodiment of the divine in the most fragile and humble form of a vulnerable infant. Not just any infant. One who wasn't above using a livestock feeding trough for a crib. ("Manger" derives from the Latin verb "to devour." What a notion, considering what was in store for that child.) Unpack that for a little while, and we discover that so much about Christianity is right there in that image:

> The King of Kings lay thus in lowly manger;
> In all our trial born to be our friend.
> He knows our need, to our weakness no stranger.

And, of course, there's some encouragement toward the end of the song, and a reminder of the message of hope:

> Truly He taught us to love one another;
> His law is love and His gospel is peace.
> Chains shall He break for the slave is our brother;
> And in His name all oppression shall cease.

It's notable that the lines about breaking chains and ending oppression are written in the future tense—which suggests there's still work to be done, and we have the potential for a better world still before us.

Lyric analysis aside, part of why this song is so important to me is that becoming a father has been, for me, the clearest and most unambiguous affirmation of my worth and purpose before God. Holding a new life, so full of possibility, is a profound and humbling celebration of hope. The whole "savior as an infant" thing suddenly makes total, perfect, and holy sense. That's what Christianity holds at its core: We are loved equally, and yet paradoxically beyond measure, by God—like a parent.

We exist because we are loved.

And we are loved because we exist.

A Foundation for Justice

The second thing I believe because of my faith is predicated on the first: If we are all indeed loved children of God, brothers and sisters in and of Christ, then we should treat each other accordingly. I'm not sure what better foundation for justice, love, and care there could be.

We need that, because life is hard, and we don't all get along all the time. Trying to live a life of this faith is a constant challenge that goes like this: "Well, you're really screwed up and driving me nuts. But hey, after all, we are all loved children of the divine creator of the universe. So, um, I guess you're actually kind of a big deal, and so am I, even though I'm pretty screwed up in my own ways too, and even though I drive you nuts, too. So, I guess we owe it to each other to love one another."

This struggle reminds me of growing up with my four brothers, each of us driving each other nuts and our exasperated parents reminding us that we were worthy and deserving of each other's love, patience, and forgiveness. The Gospel of John tells us about that oh-so-important command to love one another. Jesus isn't making a casual suggestion. It isn't, "Hey, guys. When and if you have time, maybe think about loving one another as I have loved you, okay?" No. The key word is "command." The quote goes like this: "This I command you: Love one another as I have loved you" (John 13:34–35).

So, I find this "you're all brothers and sisters" message of Christianity to be an accessible, honest, relatable, and productive way to tackle the challenges of living with other humans. That's my attempt at a concise explanation of my faith. Again, though, I'd like to think I've been doing that in many other ways throughout this book.

SPIRITUAL BUT NOT RELIGIOUS?

Okay, so I've got my faith. Good for me. Why should you embrace a religious faith tradition? I hear this all the time: "I'm spiritual but I'm not religious." I think this is problematic for two reasons.

First off, it implies that being spiritual and being religious are entirely separate propositions. They aren't the same thing, no. But they are intertwined. The second problem is that it implies that being spiritual isn't really a big deal.

Well, which is it? I mean, if we're spiritual—that is, if we believe that there is an aspect of our being that is beyond our biological body, then isn't that a pretty big deal? Isn't it actually *the most important thing?*

And if so, doesn't that mean you should organize your life accordingly? To attempt to understand that spiritual identity? In our short lifespan, to dedicate ourselves to preparing for whatever comes next?

That's why, when students tell me they're "spiritual but not religious," I often ask, "Well, why do you consider yourself spiritual?" Usually, the response is a variation on this: "Well, I believe that we're more than just flesh and blood, but I don't like organized religion."

Which is totally fine. Except that it doesn't really address the problem I raised a couple paragraphs ago. If we are spiritual beings, man, then *we are a really big deal.* Maybe, just maybe, the centuries—no, millennia—of fellow humans who came before us, spending their lifetimes wrestling with life's biggest existential questions, just like we do, were onto something in terms of these organized religions. Put another way—if you believe you're more than flesh and blood, doesn't it make sense to do everything you can to nurture your spiritual life? Ancient religious traditions didn't just drop out of the sky. They're time-tested, ancient modes of being that have endured an awful lot of human experience. They offer time-tested frameworks for living—the kind of frameworks that help us form a telos.

They provide something unmoving to fall back on.

They provide a foundation of principles and ethics.

Yes, you might take issue with a few, or maybe even many, of the teachings. Yes, you might find yourself wildly opposed to certain doctrines, stances, or policies. Yes, you might be disgusted by scandal and hypocrisy perpetrated by some. Fair points, all. But they don't negate the value of having a baseline set of principles that guide ethical behavior and hold you to unmoving standards.

Human life is messy, which is why faith traditions include elements and means of redemption, renewal, and reconciliation. Remember, those ancient traditions didn't get to be ancient by ignoring human nature. If you haven't considered investing yourself in a religious faith tradition, maybe give it some thought. Or, if you've become disillusioned with your religion, maybe it's worth a reboot. Maybe in a different place, with different people.

Religious practice helps us discern a telos. It can bring discipline, balance, and direction to a young guy's life. It can also bring joy, hope, encouragement, and optimism.

Companionship for the Long Haul

I often question what I believe. When things are in really bad shape—on bad days, weeks, months, or even years, like the ones after I quit the Academy—those doubts almost take over.

But somehow, something deep in my core hangs on and keeps me going. It's times like that, when I'm feeling most alone and desolate, that the loving companionship of Jesus—a guy who knew suffering—is most apparent. I suppose that's the main reason why I wear a cross on the silver chain around my neck. It's a reminder.

My religious tradition helps me navigate the path, especially during the hardest parts. Sometimes I regret that I'm not as attentive to my faith life as I should be when the way is smooth. But there's no denying that it's been crucial to me when the path is at its most rugged. Whenever we've experienced a death in the family, for example, I've found myself consciously grateful for the faith tradition that binds us together. Sure, we can take issue with religious institutions. Sure, we can roll our eyes at certain things or find weekly obligations tedious. But I'll tell you what: at these moments when things seem at their most tenuous, everyone knows where to go and what to expect in this big Catholic family. There will be a funeral. There will be a Mass. There will be prayers at a burial. It will matter. There will be an overarching conviction—held among people with varied levels of skepticism, doubt, belief, and religious practice—that someone we spent a lifetime loving has not simply ceased to exist with the cessation of cardiac rhythms.

That's a deeply powerful thing to have and hold on to at these tough junctures. I often wonder how much harder it must be for people who have no such framework to find peace and consolation in these moments.

—⁓—

Winter hiking can be beautiful—as long as the weather is good. Almost fifteen years ago, I did a camping trip in the Adirondacks with a couple of friends. We had clear blue skies, and the crystal-white snow glistened brightly even through the sunglasses that shielded our eyes from the glare. The air was still and silent except for the crunch of our crampon-spiked boots and our labored breathing as the three of us clambered up the snow-covered trail toward the peak.

The view from the top was stunning, and without the slightest puff of wind, it was warm enough to shed layers. We took pictures in our T-shirts and snow pants, and spent a good hour enjoying the panorama, not another soul in sight.

It was a long but beautiful hike back to the campground, where our site was nestled near the shore of a small frozen lake. The icy expanse glowed with blue-white moonlight under a pitch-black, starry sky.

We were still warm from exertion as we set up our tents and started our stove to make dinner. We knew it wouldn't be long before our body heat faded, though, so we got busy building a fire. We took our time and did it right, ensuring it was well-built. Soon, there was a small but steady fire burning, the center of it a pile of red-hot embers.

Within an hour, a front moved in and began dropping dense, heavy snowflakes that piled up quickly. But our small fire held up, despite the snow that fell on it. The heart of the fire remained strong, radiating a circle of heat that staved off the bitter chill. We were able to sit around it for hours, even as snow piled up around us. We had some good laughs. But we also talked about some serious stuff. One of us was dealing with something heavy, and because of this, that conversation around the fire was pretty important.

We weren't deep in the wilderness. We were at a campground. So our fire wasn't a matter of survival. Not that time, anyway. It usually isn't. But if that fire hadn't endured—if the circle of warmth hadn't been there—we would have just zipped into our tents and sleeping bags and gone to sleep. We wouldn't have had that important conversation.

The heart of the fire was strong. It kept us in each other's company. It ushered forth honesty. And it saw us through a dark winter night.

That's the case for faith, guys. It can see us through the darkness. And it can equip us with what we need to help others through it, too.

"The light shines in the darkness, and the darkness has not overcome it" (John 1:5).

Epilogue
Parting Words

As I MENTIONED, the Jesuits have taught me to begin and end with gratitude. This book began with a dedication—an expression of thanks. I want to end it with an expression of gratitude to you.

When you write a book, you have no way of knowing who will read it, or when, or under what circumstances. You imagine that someday, maybe in the next year or two, while you're doing something mundane like washing the dishes or making a sandwich or working at your computer, someone somewhere will be reading what you wrote. And, of course, you'll have no idea.

You also realize that your book will be around longer than you will, and maybe decades from now, after you've moved on from this mortal life, someone who isn't even born yet might find an old copy on a shelf, dust it off, and read it. When you think of it like that, publishing a book is sort of like shining a flashlight beam up into the starry sky, knowing that light is now traveling far and fast, to places you'll never know or see. It's really humbling.

I'm smiling as I write these closing words, because I'm picturing you reading them, wherever and whoever you are. I don't know you. I don't know where you're from, or what color your skin is, or what your family looks like, or what you believe, or who you're attracted to, or what you aspire to do with your life. I don't know your personality or your politics. I don't know if you're lonely as hell, or deeply in love with someone, or maybe both.

I just see a young guy full of potential and full of life, who maybe has struggled in some of the same ways I have, who perhaps has wrestled with some of the same difficult questions, who has sometimes also found himself desolate and discouraged. Maybe you're still very young, and you're just starting out thinking about what to build with your life. Maybe you've built something but aren't sure it's what you really wanted to build, after all. Maybe you've built a tower that has become unstable and has fallen over, or seems like it's about to. Whatever your case may be, I picture you now, reading these final paragraphs, hopefully feeling just a little bit stronger and more encouraged as you walk your path. That image brings me joy.

The idea that these reflections may have helped or encouraged you, even just a little, is a gift to me. That maybe, reading this has been a reminder to you that you are loved despite your messiness—and that to be a bit of a mess is a natural, normal part of being human. That you matter, and that so much potential and possibility lies ahead on the path before you. The thought that what I've written here might make even a small positive difference in your life is a gift to me, as a writer, as a teacher, and simply as a fellow man. If this book has likewise been a gift to you, I hope you might share it with someone else who could also use some encouragement. Many other guys could use some. I'm sure of it. They just might not say it. It's hard to ask for help.

Thank you for walking with me for a while. As our paths diverge, I'll leave you with this:

The world needs good men.

Your life is a gift and an opportunity.

So get up early, get out there, be honest, and work hard at what is good.

Keep going on your path, with courage, humility, kindness, and hope.

You matter.

Notes

Chapter 1. Making Your Path

1. Machado, A. *Border of a Dream.* Port Townsend, WA: Copper Canyon Press, 2004.

2. Peterson, Jordan B. *12 Rules for Life: An Antidote to Chaos.* London: Penguin, 2019.

3. Tolkien, J. R. R. *The Fellowship of the Ring: Being the First Part of The Lord of the Rings.* Boston: Mariner Books/Houghton Mifflin Harcourt, 2012.

4. Frankl, Viktor. *Man's Search for Meaning.* Boston, MA: Beacon Press, 2006.

Chapter 2. Not a Straight Line

1. Fleming, David, SJ. *What Is Ignatian Spirituality?* Chicago: Loyola Press, 2008.

Chapter 3. Getting to Virtue

1. Roy, Michael M., and Liersch, Michael J. "I Am a Better Driver Than You Think: Examining Self-Enhancement for Driving Ability." *Journal of Applied Social Psychology*, 43, no. 8 (2013): 10.1111 /jasp.12117.

2. Durant, Will. *The Story of Philosophy: The Lives and Opinions of the World's Greatest Philosophers from Plato to John Dewey*. New York: Pocket Books, 1927/1991.

3. *Aristotle's Nicomachean Ethics*, translated by Bartlett, Robert C., and Collins, Susan D. Chicago: The University of Chicago Press, 2011.

Chapter 5. Life as Pilgrimage

1. Cousineau, Phil. "Prologue." In O'Reilly, Sean, and O'Reilly, James, eds. *Pilgrimage: Adventures of the Spirit* (p. xv). San Francisco: Traveler's Tales, 2000.

Chapter 6. Learning as Adventure

1. Reeves, Richard, and Smith, Ember. "Boys Left Behind: Education Gender Gaps Across the US." Brookings Institute. October 12, 2022. https://www.brookings.edu/articles/boys-left-behind-education-gender-gaps-across-the-us/.

2. Klein, Ezra. "The Men—and Boys—Are Not Alright." The Ezra Klein Show. March 10, 2023. https://www.nytimes.com/2023/03/10/opinion/ezra-klein-podcast-richard-reeves.html.

3. National Center for Education Statistics, a component of the US Department of Education and the Institute of Education Sciences. "Digest of Education Statistics—Table 303.70: Total Undergraduate Fall Enrollment in Degree-Granting Postsecondary Institutions, by Attendance Status, Sex of Student, and Control and Level of Institution: Selected Years, 1970 through 2031. https://nces.ed.gov/programs/digest/d22/tables/dt22_303.70.asp.

4. Park, Mina, and Schmidt, Milena. "Trends in Consumer Book Buying [Infographic]." Penguin Random House News for

Authors. June 2013. http://authornews.penguinrandomhouse.com /trends-in-consumer-book-buying-infographic/.

5. Perrin, Andrew. "Book Reading 2016." Pew Research Center. September 1, 2016. https://www.pewresearch.org/internet/2016 /09/01/book-reading-2016/.

6. Reeves, Richard, and Secker, Will. "We Need More Apprenticeships." American Institute for Boys and Men. November 10, 2023. https://aibm.org/commentary/apprenticeships/.

Chapter 7. Telos: Developing a Life Vision

1. Covey, Stephen. *The 7 Habits of Highly Effective People.* New York: Free Press, 1989.

2. McTighe, Jay, and Wiggins, Grant. *Understanding by Design.* Alexandria, VA: Association for Supervision and Curriculum Development, 2005.

Chapter 9. The Integrated Man

1. Gurian, Michael. "The Case for Gender Difference." The Gurian Institute. April 11, 2019. https://gurianinstitute.com/amaz ing-evidence-of-female-and-male-brains/.

2. Ryali, Srikanth, Zhang, Yuan, de los Angeles, Carlo, Supekar, Kaustubh, and Menon, Vinod. "Deep Learning Models Reveal Replicable, Generalizable, and Behaviorally Relevant Sex Differences in Human Functional Brain Organization." *Proceedings of the National Academy of Sciences.* February 20, 2024. https://www.pnas.org/doi/10 .1073/pnas.2310012121.

3. Gurian, Michael. *The Wonder of Boys* (tenth anniversary edition). New York: TarcherPerigree, 2006.

Chapter 10. Traveling Companions

1. Garnett, Matthew F., Curtin, Sally C., and Stone, Deborah M. "Suicide Mortality in the United States, 2000–2020." NCHS Data Brief 433. Hyattsville, MD: National Center for Health Statistics, 2022.

Chapter 11. Machine Maintenance

1. Jargon, Julia. "Screens, Lack of Sun Are Causing an Epidemic of Myopia." *The Wall Street Journal.* August 26, 2023. https://www.wsj .com/tech/personal-tech/our-eyes-really-are-getting-worse-heres -how-to-save-your-kids-vision-de16d592.

Chapter 12. Service and Leadership

1. Lanza, Kevin, Hunt, Ethan T., Mantey, Dale S., Omega-Njemnobi, Onyinye, Cristol, Benjamin, and Kelder, Stephen H. "Volunteering, Health, and Well-Being of Children and Adolescents in the United States." *JAMA Netw Open*, 6, no. 5 (2023): e2315980.

2. Park, Soyoung Q., et al. "A Neural Link between Generosity and Happiness." *Nat. Commun.* 8 (2017): 15964.

Chapter 13. Wired Up

1. Abbey, Edward. *Desert Solitaire: A Season in the Wilderness.* New York: Simon & Schuster, 1990.

Chapter 14. Hormones and Habits

1. Robbins, Cynthia L., Schick, Vanessa, Reece, Michael, et al. "Prevalence, Frequency, and Associations of Masturbation with Part-

nered Sexual Behaviors Among US Adolescents." *Arch Pediatr Adolesc Med*, 165, no. 12 (2011): 1087–93.

2. https://www.fightthenewdrug.org.

3. Wright, Paul J., Paul, Bryant, and Herbenick, Debby. "Preliminary Insights from a U.S. Probability Sample on Adolescents' Pornography Exposure, Media Psychology, and Sexual Aggression." *J. Health Commun.*, 26, no. 1 (2021): 39–46.

4. Lim, Megan S. C., Agius, Paul A., Carrotte, Elise R., Vella, Alyce M., and Hellard, Margaret E. "Young Australians' Use of Pornography and Associations with Sexual Risk Behaviours." *Australian and New Zealand Journal of Public Health*, 41, no. 4 (2017): 438–43.

5. Love, Todd, Laier, Christian, Brand, Matthias, Hatch, Linda, and Hajela, Raju. (2015). "Neuroscience of Internet Pornography Addiction: A Review and Update." *Behavioral Sciences* (Basel, Switzerland), 5(3): 388–433.

CHAPTER 15. WORK, MONEY, AND FREEDOM

1. Machado, A. *Border of a Dream*. Port Townsend, WA: Copper Canyon Press, 2004.

2. Kahneman, Daniel, and Deaton, Angus. "High Income Improves Evaluation of Life but Not Emotional Well-Being." *Psychological and Cognitive Sciences*, 107, no. 38 (2010).

3. Killingsworth, Matthew A. "Experienced Well-Being Rises with Income, Even Above $75,000 per Year." *Proceedings of the National Academy of Sciences*, 118, no. 4 (2021).

4. Killingsworth, Matthew A., Kahneman, Daniel, and Mellers, Barbara. "Income and Emotional Well-Being: A Conflict Resolved." *Proceedings of the National Academy of Sciences*, 120, no. 10 (2023).

Chapter 17. A Case for Faith

1. Cumbo, Paul. "Joy Rekindles Faith at a Family Wedding." *The Buffalo News*. September 15, 2019.

2. Dwight, John Sullivan. "Oh Holy Night." 1955 English translation of "Minuit Chrétiens" by Cappeau, Placide (1847).

Acknowledgments

I'm a storyteller at heart, and fiction is my comfort zone. Writing a book like this is a whole different animal, though, and I needed help. I owe a debt of gratitude to Michael Gurian, whose editorial advice was key both in terms of content, structure, and expression. His expertise is cited explicitly; however, his influence no doubt permeates much of what I've written. Dr. Rajeev Ramchand, an expert in adolescent development, offered a helpful critical read early on. My dad, Dr. Tom Cumbo, provided both a sharp line edit and numerous insights gleaned from a lifetime of raising five sons. Other prominent experts with whom I've had the pleasure to connect have helped me come to understand these things over the years through their research, writing, and presentations. These include Dr. Jordan Peterson, Dr. Leonard Sax, Dr. Michael Reichert, Dr. Richard V. Reeves, and Dr. James Power.

I'm grateful to some more casual readers whose insights on various drafts were helpful, including Sean O'Neill, Noah Lemoine, Tim Sardinia, Scott Flaherty, Rev. Jim Van Dyke, SJ, Rev. David Ciancimino, SJ, and of course my sainted mother, Anne Cumbo, who lent her nursing and counseling expertise along with the invaluable wisdom earned from raising five sons. My friend, colleague, and business partner Adam Baber has been instrumental in much of the experience that has helped me understand this stuff—and he's the guy I've done the most traveling with, by a long shot. I'm indebted to Tom Flaherty, my high school coach and mentor. He hired me as a coach at age eighteen and started me building bridges. I need to thank my brother Tom and our good friend D.J. Radder, for reasons that should be clear to anyone who's read this book. I'm grateful for the kind, enthusiastic support of Luke Russert, a fellow pilgrim traveler and writer who wrote the foreword. He shares well-known and deep family ties to both Canisius High School and to the Buffalo area. (Go Bills!)

I want to thank two people important to my brief experience in the Coast Guard. Brust Roethler, my platoon leader at the Academy Introduction Mission, endorsed my admission as a cadet and gave me one of his shoulder boards as a token of affirmation. The encouragement resonated, and I still have that shoulder board. He went on to a long career as a US Coast Guard pilot. Msgr. William Cuddy, a retired Navy captain, was chaplain at the Academy. I'm grateful for the guidance he provided to a young man confronted with a difficult decision— what I now recognize was a discernment process.

Pedro Antonio Plasencia, who goes by Rafael, is one of my dearest friends and most important mentors. We met in January 2002 on my first trip to the Dominican Republic, and over the course of more than two decades, he's been a constant source of wisdom, encouragement, and tireless commitment to the shared work we've undertaken. We've collaborated on the construction of three bridges, two aqueducts, several road improvements, and at least a dozen smaller efforts to assist families and communities in need. His patience, humor, and faith have been a gift to me and many others.

I'd like to thank Jake Bonar at North Country Books for his enthusiastic interest in the manuscript, along with the editorial and marketing teams across Globe Pequot, especially Mary Wheelehan, who was helpful and patient throughout the editorial process. Likewise, I am grateful to my agent, Sheryl Shade of Shade Global, Inc., who helped this thing make it into the world—even though, you know, guys don't read books.

This book is dedicated to my brother Tom, but all four of my brothers deserve my gratitude. They were my first friends, and each of them has, in his own way, taught me a great deal about how to be a son, brother, father, husband, and human being.

Speaking of which, a guy who writes a book while also being a husband and father has to thank his wife and kids in a special way. Some of the time, energy, and investment that goes into a book comes at their expense. I can only hope that the end product can prove be a gift in some form to Megan, Matt, Kate, and Ben.

About the Author

Paul Cumbo has worked at Jesuit high schools for boys for more than twenty years, mostly as an English teacher. He coached rowing for much of that time, and his teams have earned multiple US and Canadian national championship titles. He has written several other books and articles. His editorial services company, PJC Editorial, has a client list including some of the world's most prominent names in the corporate, academic, and nonprofit sectors. He cofounded the Camino Institute, which offers immersive, service-oriented retreats in the rural Dominican Republic. Paul lives near Buffalo, New York, with his wife and children. He is represented by his agent, Sheryl Shade, of Shade Global, Inc.

You can visit www.paulcumbo.com to learn more about Paul's other books, and subscribe to his Substack to read his shorter-form writing: paulcumbo.substack.com.